Gender and Sexuality in India

W0230211

India has one of the highest numbers of HIV carriers in the world. HIV has remained associated with sex work, and large sums of money provided to fund public health interventions have come from global institutions such as UNAIDS, the World Bank and USAID. In the midst of these processes, however, sex workers and their everyday lives have been hidden behind the rhetorics of control and prevention.

This book offers a detailed analysis of the experiences of sex workers in Chennai. Based on ethnographic fieldwork, it draws out themes of agency, notions of gender and sexuality, and the HIV prevention industry. While the women's experiences are closely knit into the medical discourse regarding sex workers, sex work emerges as a complicated knot of poverty, desire, women's oppression, love, co-option and motherhood. The author examines how the sex workers actively negotiate the risks of their industry and suggests alternative discourses on women's sexuality, sexual behaviour and desire, arguing that unless the power imbalances affecting women are addressed, such policies and activities will have little impact. She brings attention to the problems of current policies, discourses and attitudes regarding HIV, sexuality and sex work, and shows how new policies could help to reduce vulnerabilities not only for sex workers, but perhaps for all women in India.

Salla Sariola is a research associate in the Department of Anthropology at the University of Durham. Currently researching international medical research collaboration, bioethics and governance of clinical trials in Sri Lanka, her research interests include anthropology of science and technology, global health, and gender and sexuality.

Routledge/Edinburgh South Asian Studies Series

Edited by Crispin Bates and the Editorial Committee of the Centre for South Asian Studies, Edinburgh University, UK

The *Routledge/Edinburgh South Asian Studies Series* is published in association with the Centre for South Asian Studies, Edinburgh University – one of the leading centres for South Asian Studies in the UK, with a strong interdisciplinary focus. This series presents research monographs and high-quality edited volumes, as well as textbooks on topics concerning the Indian subcontinent from the modern period to contemporary times. It aims to advance understanding of the key issues in the study of South Asia, and contributions include works by experts in the social sciences and the humanities. In accordance with the academic traditions of Edinburgh, we particularly welcome submissions that emphasise the social in South Asian history, politics, sociology and anthropology, based upon thick description of empirical reality, generalised to provide original and broadly applicable conclusions.

The series welcomes new submissions from young researchers as well as established scholars working on South Asia, from any disciplinary perspective.

1   **Gender and Sexuality in India**
    Selling sex in Chennai
    Salla Sariola

Gender and Sexuality in India
Selling sex in Chennai

Salla Sariola

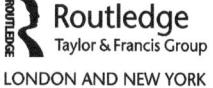
Routledge
Taylor & Francis Group

LONDON AND NEW YORK

First published 2010
by Routledge
2 Park Square, Milton Park, Abingdon, Oxon OX14 4RN

Simultaneously published in the USA and Canada
by Routledge
711 Third Ave, New York, NY 10017

*Routledge is an imprint of the Taylor & Francis Group, an informa
business*
First issued in paperback 2012

Typeset in Times New Roman by Prepress Projects Ltd, Perth, UK

British Library Cataloguing in Publication Data
A catalogue record for this book is available from the British
Library

Library of Congress Cataloging in Publication Data
Sariola, Salla. Gender and sexuality in India: selling sex in
Chennai / Salla Sariola. p. cm. — (Routledge/Edinburgh South
Asian studies series) Includes bibliographical references and
index. 1. Prostitution—India—Madras. 2. Women—Social
conditions—India—Madras. I. Title. HQ240.C44S27
2009306.740954'82—dc222009023874

ISBN13: 978-0-415-54915-8 (hbk)
ISBN13: 978-0-203-86353-4 (ebk)
ISBN13: 978-0-415-53356-0 (pbk)

Contents

Acknowledgements

I would like to thank the following people for aiding the process of this book. This book has grown out of my PhD thesis and I would like to thank my supervisory alter egos Dr Hugo Gorringe and Professor Roger Jeffery for guidance and always being there when I needed support.

Moreover, I would like to express my gratitude to Crispin Bates, the editor of the series, and Dorothea Schaefter and Suzanne Richardson, the editors at Routledge.

I would like to acknowledge the sources of funding for my PhD and thank the Economic and Social Research Council (ERSC) UK, the George Scott Travelling Scholarship, the William Dickson Travelling Fund, the Tweedie Exploration Fellowship Fund, the Society for South Asian Studies and Funds for Women Graduates.

Part of Chapter 4 was originally published in *Journal of South Asian Development*, Vol. 4:1. Copyright © Sage Publications India Pvt. Ltd. All rights reserved. Reproduced with the permission of the SAGE Publications India Pvt. Ltd, New Delhi copyright holders and the publishers.

I would also like to thank numerous individuals for sharing the path, especially my fieldwork research assistants, whose hard work and company were vital for the successful completion of the project; Iona, for transcribing; Jane, for editing; Graham, for proofreading; Julie, for sharing the years of writing up; Jaakko, for fieldwork; my family in Finland; and Greg, Linda and Allan, Dan, Jennifer, Fiona, Tom, Akshay, Filip and Lizzie, Manu, Riku, Scott, Andrea, Shahid, Jeevan, Angus, Meri and Drew, Liz, Ben, Rachel, Bob, and Blad, for their patience, conversations on the topic, and keeping me sane.

Most importantly, this research would not have been possible without the acceptance, friendliness and participation of the women and men in Chennai – *rumba nanri* (many thanks)!

Glossary and abbreviations

aattoo   autorikshaw
akka   older sister
aravani   person of third gender, also **hijra**
burkha   veil
che ayaiyo   dearie me
chuditar   loose tunic with loose trousers underneath
chumma   'just like that', casually
cini (field)   film industry
cool drinks   common name for aerated drinks, such as Coke, Fanta and
   Mirinda
Dalit   political term for outcaste or 'untouchable' castes, see also **Scheduled Caste**
devadasi   women who performed Hindu rituals in temples in the past,
   associated with prostitution
dupatta   scarf folded over shoulders, worn with **salwar kameez**
hijra   person of third gender, also **aravani**
jolly   joy, good mood, happiness, pleasure, orgasm
karpu   chastity, also **pattanaye**
keep   kept woman, concubine
kothi   'indigenous' term for a homosexual
kumkumum   red powder added on the forehead as a sign of respect or as
   a blessing
kuli   day labourer
lathi   bamboo stick used, for example, by the police
loop   intra-uterine device (IUD)
lunghi   men's waistcloth
meals   selection of curries and rice
Naicker   a higher caste of Telegu origin who have moved to Tamil Nadu
panthi   client, man, also **party**
party   client, also **panthi**

pattanaye   chastity, also **karpu**
petticoat   skirt worn under a sari
pottu   mark on the forehead between the eyes worn by Hindu women
purdah   seclusion of women
rowdy   hooligan
salwar kameez   loose tunic with loose trousers underneath, also **chuditar**
sambar   soupy curry
sangham   association
Scheduled Caste   group of outcaste or 'untouchable' castes, see also **Dalit**
shakti   feminine power
santhosham   happiness
thali   thread tied around the neck (by Hindu women), symbolising marriage
tiffin   snacks
vaange   come (in)
vanakkam   hello

1   Introduction

During my fieldwork in Chennai (formerly Madras), capital of Tamil Nadu in the south of India, between August 2004 and August 2005, I began to realise that I could use even the journeys to work – to the offices of non-governmental organisations (NGOs) working with commercial sex workers, or to interview some of their members and visitors – as opportunities to observe and understand what it means to be a sex worker in the city. One morning I challenge the traffic over a stinky river and get to the bus stop.

I have learned that women solicit by standing at bus stops. I look around at the women there. I know that the sex workers do not look any different from other women, so anyone could be soliciting. I look around me ... Would I be able to identify a sex worker after meeting so many? Autorikshaws drive slowly past the bus stop, offering rides. As far as I know, some autorikshaw drivers act as middlemen. I catch a man staring at me. I quickly turn my eyes away.

I am on my way to meet a sex worker for an interview. I met her a couple of months earlier at an NGO meeting. We were introduced by other sex workers, and she was keen on being interviewed for my research. First, I must collect my translator at the Vadapazhani bus depot near the film studios, near the sex worker's neighbourhood. Suddenly, while I am waiting for my translator, two women that I know walk past. They see me and stop to talk. They speak Tamil very quickly; I can understand enough to tell that they know me from the NGO. They act strangely, talk and laugh loudly and are distracted, and I realise that they are drunk. Being drunk is very rare for Tamil women, but it is a common way for sex workers to relax. It dawns on me that they have probably been seeing clients. I greet them, but after exchanging niceties in a somewhat haphazard way (the women are giggling, erratic in their conversation), they tumble away.

My translator arrives and we walk to where the sex worker lives. After our initial introduction at the NGO, we had arranged a previous meeting to which she never showed up. After bumping into her again at the NGO, she convinced me that she still wanted to talk to me; she had just been unable to be home at the previous time we had arranged. This time, she is there. She invites us in with a smile. '*Vanakkam, vanakkam! Vaange vaange!*' ('Hello, hello! Come in, come in!'). We are invited inside and sit on the floor. Her house is small, with brick walls and a thatched roof. Colourful plastic pots of water are lined up next to the wall. She has a small kerosene stove; cooking pots fill the shelves. There are pictures of dead relatives and images of gods on the wall. After polite questions regarding her family's health, her health, her children's health, and the well-being of all the people we know together, I ask how she feels about the interview. She says she's happy to talk, and I pull out the recorder. I explain to her once again about my work, and that what she tells me will be confidential and anonymous, and that I will not share her information with the NGOs. She sends a neighbour, who has come in to see what is going on, to buy some *cool drinks* for us. I ask her to tell me, in her own words, her life story. The following narrative is not based on one individual, but it is merged together from the narratives of several women whom I interviewed during my fieldwork.

Mariamma starts by recounting a normal day in her life as a sex worker. She is a woman in her late twenties and a mother of two, living in a small hut in Chennai, Tamil Nadu. On this particular day she sends the children to school, washes the dishes from the night before and prepares some rice and *sambar*, a soupy lentil curry, for the evening. She washes the children's clothes and hangs them to dry. Around noon, she gets a phone call. An older lady she knows from her neighbourhood tells her that there are clients who would pay for sex, if she was interested. (The lady is her madam, an older sex worker who connects sex workers with men who want to pay for sex.) Mariamma is penniless and the ration of rice is almost gone. Her children have not eaten anything else but the thin *sambar* that whole week. Her son, in particular, has had a cough for a long time. Mariamma is worried. The lady on the phone tells her that there are two men waiting at Parry's Corner, a big bus depot. Mariamma says yes and rushes to call her friend Sarasvati, who agrees to come along. (Mariamma and Sarasvati like to work together; it provides them with security and makes them feel less alone. They have been friends for a long time and they know everything about each other. They always go to meet clients together – about three times a week.)

Mariamma gets dressed for her work. She changes from her nightgown into a *sari*. She puts on a bright red bra underneath. She has three *saris* hanging from a string on the wall. They are all made of cheap, artificial material: one yellow, one blue and one red. She chooses the yellow one and folds it around her. She searches for her red lipstick; she has hidden it away from the children in the far end corner of her cupboard. She sees herself from a cracked piece of mirror, applies lipstick on her lips and rubs it on her cheeks as well. Finally, she brushes her long hair and plaits it. To please the clients, she wants to look beautiful – but not too flashy: she does not want to draw too much attention to herself. She is afraid that someone might recognise her and realise what she is doing. She is afraid for her own and her children's reputation. If she were caught then everybody would come to know. She is sure that she would then have to move house again and her children would be thrown out of their school. It has happened to others.

Mariamma walks through the area she lives in – a slum area that has been improved a little by a local NGO. The neighbourhood has concrete houses and water pumps at the ends of the roads. The water truck comes twice a week to fill up the water tanks, but even so it is not enough for everybody for the whole week. Most of the houses are similar, with two floors, with families from different backgrounds living together. Within the houses, the flats are small, around three by three metres each, with a small kitchen space and a communal toilet. The narrow roads are just wide enough to drive an *aattoo* (autorikshaw) through; they are covered with broken and crumbled concrete. It takes about 20 minutes for Mariamma to walk from her house to the main road and the bus stop. It is hot and she is sweating, but she cannot afford to take an autorikshaw every time. She meets Sarasvati at the main junction, they buy plenty of flowers to put into their hair and then catch a bus to Parry's Corner.

At Parry's Corner, it takes them a long time to find the men. Parry's Corner is a big bus depot: hundreds of buses depart daily to take people to the neighbourhoods of Chennai. While the women search for the men, two policemen patrol the area. Mariamma freezes; she is afraid of the police. She has experienced what it means to be caught at the bus stop and questioned. Other women have also told her that the policemen at the station demand money, and that they force women to have sex with them. The two women stand on a platform and pretend that they are waiting for a bus until the policemen have gone.

Finally, they use their mobile phone to call the clients: they are standing next to a fruit vendor. The four of them greet like people who know each other well, to avoid attention. The men are in their mid-20s. They are dressed in white-collared shirts and straight trousers. One of them has a mobile phone hanging from his neck, tucked away in the front pocket of his shirt. They look decent, so the women decide to go with them. The men say that they will pay Rs. 500 between the two of them. Mariamma and Sarasvati agree and they all walk together to a nearby lodge.

The lodge is dirty, with faded turquoise walls, stained from the damp of many rainy seasons. Images of Hindu gods hang from the wall. The men pay Rs. 100 for the room and they all go in. The men who run the lodge know well what the room is for, but they ask no questions. The room has two small bare beds and nothing more. The sheets are dirty. Mariamma confirms that they will get Rs. 500 and clarifies that there has to be condoms.

The men have brought a bottle of whisky with them and they offer it to the women. Mariamma and Sarasvati have a drink to relax. They chat. Mariamma nearly vomits from the bitter taste of the whisky but it soothes her and she soon feels floppy. Sarasvati chats to the fatter man. Mariamma turns to take off her sari, folds it carefully and places it in the corner, now feeling vulnerable and exposed. In the meantime, Sarasvati starts to give oral sex to the fat man. Mariamma does not look. The slim man wants her to take all her clothes off – the petticoat, blouse and the red bra – but she refuses. He grabs her breasts forcefully, pulls her blouse so that it tears and shows the red bra, and throws her onto the bed. He climbs on top of her and penetrates her. By this point, Mariamma is so drunk that she has stopped worrying about anything. As soon as everything is over, the women demand the money. It turns out that the men only have Rs. 400 with them. The women protest and quarrel with the men, but as the men say they have no more, Mariamma and Sarasvati have to accept whatever they can get, and leave.

They wander off to Parry's Corner and chat. They are agitated at being cheated. Mariamma has a pounding headache and her body aches too. They stop to buy some *meals*, rice and spicy curry sauces, and take them back to Mariamma's house to eat. Sarasvati leaves and Mariamma lies down on the mat on the floor to take some rest. She falls asleep thinking of her children. She feels how much she loves them and tears fill her eyes.

The above narrative illustrates the concerns of some of the women who sell sex in India. The narrative also shows how difficult it is to research female sex workers. There is a silence – around women's sexuality, around the shame that many women experienced and risks they took by identifying themselves as sex workers – that makes it hard to engage with sex workers and truncated what they told me. The findings I report in this book are framed by these difficulties and the particular perspective that directed my questions: to analyse the lives of sex workers outwith the medicalised perspective implied in HIV prevention, the predominant public discourse where sex work is addressed in India.

Until the discovery of HIV amongst a group of sex workers deported from Mumbai to Chennai, the capital of the southern state of Tamil Nadu, in 1986, commercial sex workers hardly appeared on the public map of issues and concerns. Twenty years later, the United Nations Joint Programme on HIV/AIDS (UNAIDS) (2006) announced that India, with 5.7 million people, had the highest number of HIV carriers in the world. The association between sex work and HIV that characterised the start of the history of HIV in India has been prominent since, and HIV has remained associated with sex work more than with any other 'high-risk groups', such as homosexuals or intravenous drug users. Not surprisingly, then, many agencies – governmental as well as NGOs, national and international – have been interested in harnessing sex workers to prevent HIV. Global institutions, such as UNAIDS, the World Bank, and the United States Agency for International Development (USAID), have provided large amounts of resources to fund and organise public health interventions. While this framing of the problem of HIV has brought much needed attention to curb its spread, in the midst of these processes, sex workers and their everyday lives have been hidden from view. The rhetorics of control and prevention have dominated the debate. The argument in this book is that such a medicalised view is limited, detached from the lives of the sex workers, and can lead to very partial and misleading evidence and thus to ineffective policies.

Feminist and post-structuralist approaches to sex work

I carried out ethnographic fieldwork in Chennai, Tamil Nadu, between August 2004 and August 2005. I interviewed fifty-six women, and took part in activities and interviewed staff at six NGOs that were involved in HIV prevention work. Throughout this book my concern is to describe the lives of sex workers, as far as possible, using their own words. I have been particularly alert to evidence of agency: actions, decisions and responses through which these women show how far, when and where they have been able to take some control over their lives. Without victimising or judging them, my account shows how marginalised women use power to negotiate their lives. I argue and provide evidence for how selling sex was one way of negotiating the material and discursive contexts through which the women navigated their everyday lives. Looking beyond the medicalised discourse regarding sex workers, selling sex can be seen as a complicated knot of poverty, desire, women's oppression, love, co-option, and motherhood. I do not take a stance on the wider issues of structure and agency that have fascinated and exhausted social scientists for decades, but rather provide a nuanced analysis of the power that sex workers use as individuals in seemingly powerless positions. Recently, agency has been discussed in post-structuralist feminist writings and although my analysis fits loosely into this theoretical framework, it is not an attempt to test these theories by reference to the lives of the sex workers. My methodology demands the opposite – an analysis that is strongly rooted in the data from my fieldwork and to the voices of the sex workers. Central to my use of the concept of agency is Foucault's theory of power. In his *History of Sexuality* Vol. 1, Foucault (1998 [1976]: 92–102) suggests that power exists in all relationships and is thus everywhere and ever present. The idea that this power can be used by all individuals has enabled analyses in which individuals are seen as subjects who negotiate the time- and space-specific contexts that they live in. Following this theoretical premise, throughout this book I provide evidence of how we should see sex workers – like other individuals – as individuals who are able to negotiate the conditions of oppressive discourses, structures of patriarchy and stigma on prostitution that surround them to various degrees, and not as essentialised victims.[1]

How do we understand the agency of people who seemingly have little power? How do we understand why women engage with practices that, from a liberalist viewpoint, are oppressive? One viewpoint suggests that such women might be suffering from false consciousness. According to another, women have been socialised into their own oppression (for a critique of these positions, see Mahmood 2005: 6). My position departs from these writings: rather than labelling these women as victims who are passive or unable to understand their best interest, we need to understand the ways in which human agency exists within structures of subordination, but without romanticising this activity as resistance (see, for example, Abu-Lughod 1990; Scott 1985).

The work of Saba Mahmood provides a relevant model for my approach. In the first chapter of her book on women's participation in a pious Islamic movement in Egypt, *Politics of Piety – The Islamic Revival and the Feminist Subject* (Mahmood 2005), she problematises the conceptual underpinning of feminism as a derivative of liberalist and emancipatory politics. Mahmood questions the universality of the desire to be 'free' of structures of domination and suggests that the concept of resistance has been part of a liberalist project. By discussing resistance only in the context of 'acting *against* domination', such an approach also reinforces the dichotomy of agency as *either* resistance *or* domination – leaving little or no space for anything else. Following Foucault, Mahmood argues that in order to understand power and agency properly, these issues need to be studied in their historical and cultural contexts. From a liberalist framework and without cultural contextualisation, some action might be missed or misinterpreted 'from outside'. It is overly simplistic, Mahmood argues, to look at resistance only as activity against, for example, patriarchal dominance; instead, all action should be seen as agency. This takes the analysis of power used by marginalised groups a step further. It is not only a necessary to understand how agency is enacted by people who seemingly have little power but also to recognise that there are forms of agency that do not aim at 'liberation'. Instead, agency should be understood as holistic 'activity' that includes both – at times this might mean that people make choices that are 'restricting' and 'oppressive' and at other times and places 'subversive' and 'liberating'. From Mahmood's perspective, both liberatory and oppressive forces can operate in an individual's life simultaneously. Following the same logic, my book is, therefore, a study of how oppression and agency can co-exist in the lives of sex workers in contemporary India. This book is an analysis of agency on the margins, and I explore four key themes on how the women I interviewed as part of this research used agency. I show how they understood and explained their involvement in sex work, how they benefited from their relationships with HIV prevention NGOs, how they negotiated the problems in sex work, and, finally, how they used power with regard to issues of sexuality – an area with least power for women in Indian society.

The developing argument

Sex workers are some of the most vulnerable people in India today, and the violent realities of sex workers' lives are undeniable. The women I interviewed lived in oppressive contexts where jobs for women are rare, poor women are often forced to take sole responsibility for children, and they may have few other family contacts. All of these issues affect the lives of other poor women: in addition, as sex workers, the women I met were vulnerable to violence by police and clients. These women were also frequently ostracised by their families, and many lived in fear of spoiling the reputations of their children. Many of them had internalised the stigma surrounding sex work to the extent that they dreaded the sex work they did. Furthermore, their ability to negotiate the use of condoms was limited: they are in an inferior social position in all domains of power in the client encounter – in terms of gender, money and their disrespected role as a sex worker – which makes them constantly vulnerable to sexually transmitted diseases (HIV and STDs). Nevertheless, these women were still able to make choices and act on their own account, both on a daily basis and in the long term. They negotiated performing sex in ways that were least harmful to them, physically and mentally, and that were the least harmful to their reputation.

Such a viewpoint – one that recognises that women in sex work can have agency and/or are not just victims of their surroundings – has informed some existing academic debates of sex work (predominantly originating from the global North), particularly over whether selling sex is work or essentially violence against women. This viewpoint rejects the abolitionist stance to prostitution (for example, Barry 1984; Jeffreys 1997) according to which women who sell sex are victims of the power relations between men and women. Sex workers' movements argue that selling sex is work and that women have the right to do with their bodies what they want, including selling sex (see, for example, Nagle 1997; Pheterson and St James 1989). This notion that women can have agency in selling sex has enabled analyses of sex work that are nuanced, and complicated by the experiences of women themselves (see for example Brevis and Linstead 2000a,b; Day 2007; Nencel 2001; Sanders 2005a,b; Wardlow 2006; Zatz 1997). Like these writers, I argue that a properly contextualised, culturally specific analysis is needed, rather than relying on universalist conceptions of the nature of selling sex. So, Chapter 2 describes Chennai, India, with regard to gender, sexuality and HIV. This chapter provides the conceptual and material context for the subsequent chapters, which present aspects of sex workers' own accounts of their lives and of those who deal with them – especially the HIV control agencies.

In the following chapters, I ask you, the reader, to join me in seeing these women as they presented themselves: not as victims of their conditions, but as agentive women who use selling sex to serve their interests. The ethnographic chapters (Chapters 3–6) show how, for these women, selling sex was a way to obtain money and a better financial future for themselves and their children. But it also offered further chances: of access to love, intimacy and desire, and even, in some cases, roles in films. These women provide insights into how even the poorest and apparently most downtrodden women are able to 'make out'. Selling sex involved relative and personal negotiation, and Chapter 3 illustrates this process through women's in-depth life stories.

Chapter 4 analyses how the women were involved in HIV prevention activities. HIV is the main public arena in which sex work in India has been discussed. The attention has been limited to HIV as a health problem and I argue that sex work is discussed in this public discourse as an epidemiological category. HIV prevention offers a particular subject position to sex workers, some of whom chose to take part in it and thus reinforce it. Sex workers in Chennai used the HIV prevention NGOs for making financial gains through peer education and (ab)using incentives for participating in meetings arranged by these organisations. Peer education, generating HIV awareness, provided an opportunity to negotiate and subvert the stigma of sex work with a more positive identity – that of someone active in HIV prevention. However, despite some sex-working women's participation in HIV prevention programmes the official representation is a simplification of the realities of the sex workers. Looking at women from a more socially orientated point of view – one that is informed by feminist theories of gender and sexuality – brings sex workers to life, showing them as far more than the limited HIV representation can envisage. Moreover, a social analysis that extends beyond the context of HIV as a health problem to (gender) inequalities in the wider Indian society brings out problems in the existing HIV prevention policies. Unless the power imbalances created by patriarchal structures that affect all women are addressed, HIV prevention activities will continue to have little real impact. Nevertheless, the women's engagement with the HIV prevention NGOs represents another form of agency that women used as an alternative source of funds as well as gaining a positive social role.

The dominant discourse of women in India portrays a rigid role for them: as reproductive, self-sacrificing mothers for whom sexual relationships are restricted to marriage and monogamy. Although HIV has raised questions of sexuality and sexual practice (taboos in India) to the fore, new theorisations of sexuality have focused on men who have sex with men rather than women who sell sex. Chapters 5 and 6 raise the question of how to understand women's selling of sex within this context. Chapter 5 describes the problems that women have faced and how they negotiated them. This chapter also describes what happens in the sex-working encounter and brings the relationships with men and other women to the fore. Chapter 6 elaborates on these relationships. How do the women, whose lives challenge normative discourses of gender and sexuality, feel about this? To what extent do they conform to those norms or resist them? What do the relationships and sexuality of sex-working women tell us about 'gender' and sexuality in contemporary India? Unsurprisingly, sexuality was a topic that even these women found hard to discuss. Until now, women's desire has been neglected in academic studies on gender in South Asia. The existing sociological and anthropological literature locates gender and sexuality in India in the context of 'normal' (heterosexual, marital, monogamous) lives. Sex workers themselves were also concerned with issues of reproduction, long-term relationships and heterosexuality, but they did not necessarily act according to the dominant normative discourses. This book demonstrates how women experienced their sexuality amid the constraints of their local contexts. Against the representation of women only as passive and concerned about reproduction, these women were found to be coquettish, erotic, non-monogamous and, at times, non-heterosexual. Chapter 6 shows that sexuality was an important but differentiated way in which sex workers deployed agency as they negotiated all of their sexual relationships. They negotiated the type of sex that they offered with this backdrop of a Tamil notion of purity. Some of them viewed anything other than vaginal sex as impure, and stuck to that, whereas others saw this social code (wives cannot do 'impure sex') as the reason why many men came to sex workers – and because the men wanted it, that was exactly the repertoire that they needed to offer. Some sex-working women preferred having random clients, whereas others preferred regular clients – and often, the women started amorous and erotic relationships with their regular clients. For some women, these relationships were their primary motivation, and the money came only as a positive side-effect. My analysis contributes to the understanding of the sexual behaviour of sex workers in particular and discourses of women's sexuality in Chennai more generally.

2   Contextualising sex work in Chennai

There is no red light district in Chennai; rather, sex work takes place all across the town. Therefore, in order to write about the context of sex work in Chennai, one must describe the various people, places and ideas that contribute to the social construction of sex work there. In this chapter I discuss the Chennai's recent economic changes, due to it becoming a target for migration within Tamil Nadu (as well as from neighbouring states) and its role in Tamil Nadu's film industry. Furthermore, sex workers operate not only in geographic spaces, but also in conceptual environments; therefore, I will also consider the discourses on gender and sexuality that inform opinions and ideas about sex work in the context of Tamil Nadu.

The discourse of HIV plays a dominating role in how sex workers are characterised – association between sex work and HIV has led to the limited, health-related, definition of the concept of 'sex work' as an epidemiological category and sex workers as vectors of HIV. This narrow focus on 'sex work' and the 'sex worker' as epidemiological concepts fails to represent the social realities of sex workers and their lives. Looking at the process of how sex workers have become central to HIV prevention leads me on to a consideration of wider discourses around gender and sexuality in India and Chennai, and dominant ideas about women and sexualities; in this chapter I trace the genealogies of these ideas to the colonial era and nationalist movements that emphasised sexual purity of women. The prominence of HIV in Tamil Nadu and the counter-hegemonic narratives provided by *devadasis*[1] and sex workers challenge dominant ideas about women's sexuality and monogamy, suggesting a conceptual lacuna in academic theorisations. The last section of this chapter provides an analysis of the existing literature on sex workers in India that usually take the viewpoint of empowerment and human rights. Although this 'development approach' does consider sex work as something other than just a health threat, it fails to sufficiently disengage from the framework of HIV or discuss any other forms of agency within the sex workers' lives, thus highlighting the need for ethnographic study.

Sexual changes?

Chennai is home to about 4.2 million people (Census (India) 2001), possibly even 7 million according to more recent unofficial estimates. Its population has risen rapidly, resulting in the city becoming the fourth most populated city in India. Chennai's urban scenery is determined by billboards; the roads are chaotic and traffic laden, defined by autorikshaws and buses tilted by the weight of their passengers. Unlike in other Indian metropolises, it is still common to come across a carriage pulled by buffalos amidst the motorcycles, bicycles, and cars. But, coming from elsewhere in Tamil Nadu, Chennai will strike one as 'urbanised'. People sometimes live on the streets, and it is business as usual for flower, fruit and *tiffin* (snack) vendors on the pavement. Men and women are rigidly differentiated in dress; the *sari* is the most preferred outfit for women, whereas men use the pant-shirt (straight trousers and a collar shirt), immaculately ironed, or a *lunghi* (loin cloth folded around the waist). Young women, especially students, can be seen wearing jeans and T-shirts or the *salwar kameez* (loose trousers and a tunic with a shawl folded over the shoulders).

Since structural adjustments that were made in 1991, Chennaites have benefited from significant technological and economical advancements. Together with the cities of Bangalore in Karnataka and Mumbai in Maharastra, Chennai is the technology hub of India. Chennai's colleges produce vast numbers of engineers, some of whom end up working in the factories of global technology giants, such as Nokia, which opened its Chennai factory in 2004. Internet cafés are mushrooming throughout Chennai and its youth spend time in malls such as Alsa Mall, Spencer Plaza or Ciscon's Complex, sipping Americano coffee and sending text messages. Although the prevailing norms regarding sexuality are conservative, the new 'modern' lifestyle has changed sexual norms and dress codes among the younger generation. For the computer literate, the Internet provides an opportunity to meet other young people of opposite sex without chaperones: meeting people in chat rooms, making and maintaining amorous relationships by email and Microsoft Network (MSN), and going through marital advertisements. Internet also gives access to sexual images and pornography in a way not seen before, and more often than not internet cafés provide cubicles for private viewings. I met many middle-class youths through friends unrelated to the sex-work industry, and they sometimes interpreted their experiences using the metaphor of being 'torn between tradition and modernity'. Norms regarding meeting the opposite sex are still restricted: this creates a demand for sexual services for young men (students and others). The sex workers I got to know defined them as a regular client group. *India Today* (Visvanathan 2006), a widely read weekly news magazine that comments on social and public issues, surveyed young men's sexuality and sexual behaviour: the results suggested that forty-nine per cent of young men nationwide had bought sex.

Changing sexual norms can be observed in a few public attempts to deconstruct the taboos around sexuality and create more realistic discourses. In 2005, Kushboo, a prominent film star and actress, spoke openly in public about the need to address issues of sexuality and made a plea for safe sex. She questioned the normative demand for women's virginity in marriage and men's open expressions of their own sexual urges. However, sex and sexuality remain sensitive subjects and Kushboo's comments created an outcry; she was seen as denigrating Tamil women's morality. Vehement criticisms were voiced, demonstrations were held against her, and crowds gathered in front of her house and the office of the Tamil Film Artists Association, equipped with brooms and flip-flops (symbols of humiliation) (Anandhi 2005); her effigies were burnt and there were calls to banish her from Tamil Nadu. *The Hindu* (30 May 2007), a national newspaper printed in Chennai, reported a further example of conservative values at the brink of a cultural change in May 2007, when the Bharatiya Janata Party (BJP) state leader L. Ganesan denounced the changes in the civil society that promoted discussions of sex, stressing that the BJP was against all sex education, especially in schools. So, although sexual norms may be changing on some level, those holding conservative attitudes still hold powerful positions in society.

Chennai as a target of socio-economic transitions

As the state capital Chennai is a centre of education and is a target of migration and transportation, all of which attract people from elsewhere in Tamil Nadu and the neighbouring states. Chennai has sizeable Telegu, Malayali and Kannada minorities. Altogether 6.6 per cent of its population are migrants (more than 400,000 people), one-third of them from other states (Census (India) 2001). Some of the migrant women end up selling sex, whereas some of the men contribute to the clientele of sex workers. As well as migrants who settle there, truck drivers (whose wives stay in their original villages and cities) also contribute to the clientele of the sex workers. Train and bus stations and road sites are common venues for soliciting. In Tamil Nadu, the AIDS Prevention and Control Society (APAC) researched truck drivers and their helpers and concluded that twenty-four per cent of them had paid for sex (APAC 2005a: 19).

Because they are uprooted from the controlling monitoring of their original communities, these client groups – students, migrants and truckers – have the freedom to purchase or provide commercial sex. The consumption of alcohol often immediately precedes the buying of sex: in the study by Sivaram *et al.* (2004a) of wine shop customers, they described the men who bought sex as an equal mix of married and unmarried men, from a range of occupations, economic statuses, working in government and private jobs, students or self-employed (for example, as autorikshaw drivers and day labourers). The cost, as well as the sex worker, was often shared. Men frequently encouraged each other to have 'riskier sex' to get value for money and gave alcohol to the sex worker hoping that she would adjust to their sexual fantasies. Alcohol fuelled men's behaviour – the men said that alcohol enabled them to be more confident, experiment sexually, and enjoy sex in general. They also reported that alcohol made them more aggressive and sometimes led to violence and forcing sex workers or partners into sex.

However, there are other factors (besides the population of uprooted men) that contribute to the demand for sex work. The norms that control women's sexuality and restrict the types of sex that they can and will perform – which I will discuss later – led men to seek out types of non-normative sex, namely oral and/or anal sex from sex workers. However, as an explication of men's motives in relation to sex work is not the aim of this study; and my observations are made from the accounts of the sex workers, rather than from interviews with clients, I will not attempt to go further into men's motives in relation to purchasing sex.

Chennai is famous for its film industry. Films are immensely popular among the Tamils, and cinema theatres provide a potential marketspace for sex workers. But the relevance of the film industry to this book goes well beyond this. As elsewhere, the glamour of the film industry has lured many people who are seeking a road to fame. The film industry hires many tens of thousands of people as supporting actors, actresses and dancers: the supporting actors and actresses union alone has 100,000 members. Many sex workers were supporting actresses or working as beauticians in the film industry, and providing free sex was defined as a 'must' in order to get a job. The same madams who arranged sex contacts also worked as middle(wo)men to help women get into the film industry. Film studios are situated near Kodambakkam and Vadapazhani bus stations, and, conveniently, these are some of the areas in which many of my informants lived. They had not, however, developed into red light districts and selling sex was not restricted to these places.

The film industry is associated with power in Tamil Nadu, particularly with Tamil nationalism: film fan clubs have been analysed from the angle of political power (Dickey 1993; Rogers 2007) and film stardom has been an influential prerequisite for political careers (see, for example, Forrester 1976). Many of the most prominent politicians in Tamil Nadu have been film stars, including M. G. Ramachandran and J. Jayalalithaa. Watching films is a common pastime, and Penny Vera-Sanso (2006) argues that the film industry in Tamil Nadu is the main source of distributing nationalist ideas and discourses to the public. While in the theatre, the audience relives these experiences and comments on the events. Films not only distribute nationalist references (for an analysis of this, see Pandian 1992), but also influence public norms around gender and sexuality. Vera-Sanso (2006) goes on to argue that the dominant ideas of women's sexuality are derived from key elements in Tamil nationalist discourses, and that film can be seen as a medium for distributing these ideas. Prostitution has been portrayed in films such as *Arrangetram* (1973) and *Mahanadi* (1993). Although these two films are not sexually explicit, many blockbusters have song and dancing scenes that are. Films often flirt with the boundaries of sexuality, but always within the acceptable norms. Although, then, there are some changes in norms regarding sexuality, films play ambiguous roles – both encouraging the portrayal of sexual licence and carrying overt messages about purity and respectability for women.

Violence of development

Accessing computers and mobile phones, gallivanting in malls, consuming films and so forth, requires a certain economic status. Development in Tamil Nadu and Chennai has not affected everyone in the same way, and the gap between the well-to-do and the poor is increasing (see, for example, Kapadia 2002; Sundaram and Tendulkar 2003). For example, twenty-five per cent of Chennai's population still live in areas that are defined in the Census as slums (Census [Tamil Nadu] 2001). The processes of development are also highly gendered; Moghadam (2005) suggests that neoliberal structural adjustments occurring since the 1980s around the globe have had a particular impact on women, increasing insecurity and vulnerability among women, and leading to the feminisation of poverty. For example, while the feminisation of labour has created some jobs for poor women, work conditions for uneducated women remain appalling and undermine condition standards agreed upon by labour unions. Padmini Swaminathan (2002) provides a critical and detailed analysis of demographic factors of caste, education level, gender, work participation and urban versus rural areas in Tamil Nadu, and she concludes that gender and caste inequalities are still actively being created. Economic changes have led young Scheduled Caste women to the labour market, but this usually entails work that is unreliable and unprotected by unions and under conditions that are unhealthy or dangerous. When strict Brahmanical norms prevail, working also has detrimental effects on women's reputations, as visibility in public means that women are outside the control of their families, thus raising questions about their reputation and honour.

Much of my fieldwork was spent in slums with people for whom the Internet, malls and cafés were not an everyday reality. The women whom I got to know lived from hand to mouth while working at jobs to support themselves and their families. Swaminathan (2002) has reported that poorly educated women, in general, from Tamil Nadu enter the labour market because other income sources are not enough to support their families. Entering sex work was done under just these types of pressures: the women I interviewed were structurally already in a vulnerable position, as they had relatively little education, had entered the labour market to support their families, and had little training to access jobs that would have supported them. They used these rationales to explain why they had entered sex work, and structural reasons, such as poverty and gender subordination, were undeniably part of the 'violence of development' (as defined by Kapadia 2002) in their lives. However, poverty and gender subordination do not explain why some women enter sex work whereas others do not. With the lack of a well-functioning welfare system in India, how women understood and negotiated the constraints of gender subordination and poverty through sex work and how they felt about this is the subject of this study. In addition to 'material' spaces, these women also work in 'conceptual' spaces; the only prominent public context where sex work is discussed is that of HIV prevention NGOs.

HIV in India and Chennai

As stated before, in 2006 UNAIDS estimated that India has the highest incidence of HIV in the world, although this was contested following new research in 2007. Indeed, Steinbrook (2007) argues that epidemiological estimates for HIV from India are much less precise than those from (for example) South Africa, due to inadequate ways of collecting data and limited numbers of venues where these data are collected. Among 14- to 50-year-olds, Indian sources estimate HIV prevalence at between 0.5 and 1.5 per cent, and the spread of HIV has shown some signs of slowing. About ninety-five per cent of women and men in Tamil Nadu have heard of HIV, which is more often than people in other states. But when it comes to knowledge of the continuous use of condoms that is needed to prevent the spread of HIV, there was a huge gap in women's and men's knowledge: eighty-two per cent of men knew that continuous use of condoms reduces the risk of HIV transmission, compared with forty-two per cent of women (Steinbrook 2007). Similar findings have been reported by Pallikavadath *et al.* (2005), who suggest that in rural Tamil Nadu, while eighty-two per cent of women knew about HIV and seventy-two per cent knew that it was possible to avoid contracting it, only thirty-one per cent knew how to do so. This suggests that women are in a disadvantaged position in terms of accessing correct information about HIV, and are thus at risk of contracting HIV when men do not initiate condom use consistently. Brahme *et al.* (2005: 383) suggest that only 7.4 per cent of men visiting a sexual health clinic in Pune used condoms regularly; some of their partners were regular girlfriends/partners, which might bring the frequency with which they use condoms down, but the percentage was higher if the partner was a sex worker. Low levels of accurate knowledge among men have also been reported by APAC (2004) and Sivaram *et al.* (2005) in Chennai and Tamil Nadu, and by Arunkumar *et al.* (2004) in Kerala.

The reasons why women are generally less aware than men of HIV and STDs lies in the women's socially subordinate position, deriving from ideas about women's honour, leading to women being secluded and (for example) less likely to go to school beyond puberty. In contexts where women's sexual purity is linked to women's honour, having knowledge of HIV and condoms can be seen as openness to promiscuity, if not of evidence of loose sexual mores (Steinbrook 2007). Sadly, having less knowledge of HIV and the need for condom use in a context where nearly all women are sterilised as the main form of contraception greatly increases their risk of HIV and other infections. Because the main attention of HIV prevention activities has been on high-risk groups, especially sex workers, the risk of HIV for all women has been increased.

Efforts to curb HIV infection have established a set of institutions that involve sex workers in a mode of attempted governance and public health control. Despite the urgent need for awareness in general, but particularly for all women, how has the notion of 'sex worker' become central to HIV prevention?

Discourse of sex work as a health concern

Apart from the *devadasis* – women who performed dance and religious rituals in Hindu temples, which, at times, included sex with priests and pilgrims, and who were deemed as prostitutes – very little literature exists on sex work in India prior to the HIV epidemic. The lack of literature up to the finding of the first infection of HIV in Chennai in 1986 suggests that sex work prior to this was largely underground – particularly after the banning of the institution of *devadasis* in the 1950s – and that it was ignored, tolerated while it remained invisible, and academically unrecognised. There were few academic accounts of sex work prior to my fieldwork, even although Venkataramana and Sarada (2001) found evidence of between 1 million and 16 million sex workers in India in 1999. This huge range in itself confirms how little accurate knowledge, particularly knowledge that is not already and misleadingly tainted by moral judgements, is available.

In India, the genealogy of the concept of 'sex worker', apart from the *devadasis*, has emerged from, and along with, the discourse of HIV. The connection made between HIV and sex work has been visible since the beginning of the epidemic and has fed into an approach by which sex workers are seen as central figures in HIV prevention, an approach influenced by guidelines of UNAIDS and the World Bank. Heterosexual contact with sex workers is seen as the reason for eighty-five per cent of HIV infections according to the National AIDS Control Organisation (NACO), the Indian government board that administers HIV prevention (NACO 2004: 14). Sex workers are defined as members of the 'high-risk group', who are at risk of being infected by HIV themselves and of transmitting it to others. The concern over HIV has brought the subject of sex work to public and academic interest, creating a plethora of writings on HIV prevention initiatives that focus on working through sex workers (see, for example, Asthana and Oostvogels 1996; Blanchard *et al.* 2005; Evans and Lambert 1997; Evans 1998; Jayasree 2004; Nag 2001; O'Neil *et al.* 2004; Pardasani 2005; Rao *et al.* 2003). Although there was hardly anything written on sex workers beforehand, since the onset of HIV nearly all academic articles on sex work have focused on the most effective prevention models, positioning sex workers as key actors. Of course sex work occurred prior to it being reported on, but the process of social construction of sex work through HIV prevention policies can nevertheless be seen as an example of how discourses 'create' social phenomena.

Most of the literature on HIV and health neglects social aspects related to sex work. As one example, among many, the work of Blanchard *et al.* (2005) demonstrates this very well. They compare the socio-demographic characteristics of 414 *devadasi* women and 1,174 other sex workers in Karnataka in relation to HIV prevention policy implications. They concluded that *devadasi* women tended to start sex work at a younger age, were more often from a rural background, were more likely to be illiterate, worked more often within their homes, and were less likely to report client violence or police harassment (Blanchard *et al.* 2005: 139). They note that this last point might be due to the 'religious' status of the *devadasi*, as well as their rootedness in rural communities where people know each other, so that if they work from home they might be less visible to 'random' and potentially violent clients and police. Blanchard *et al.* also conclude that although elsewhere in India sex workers' movements have been hampered by reluctance to identify as a sex worker, '*devadasi-hood*' could form a good basis for political movement due to a lower level of stigmatisation and a higher level of acceptance in their communities (Blanchard *et al.* 2005: 145). Their findings are fascinating but their research is carried out only in the context of HIV prevention. Because it sticks to the health policy concerns, the article misses an opportunity to analyse (for example) gender relations, 'occupational dynamics', individual experiences and meanings, whether or not there is a counter-hegemonic discourse of sexuality, points of resistance, economic relationships in sex work, sexual spaces, power dimensions, etc. Research, such as, by Blanchard *et al.* (2005) ends up reinforcing the epidemiological nature of the concept of sex worker and maintaining a very restricted stereotype of sex workers at the centre of attention in curbing the spread of HIV.

The idea that sex workers alone transmit diseases is not new. For example, in the late nineteenth century, *devadasis* and other women were made available to the British and other soldiers in the Madras compound (Raj 1993). The institution of sex work was regulated, and British officials demanded that these women should undergo regular check-ups for STDs. If they were found to be infected, they had to leave and submit to treatment and 'rehabilitation'. The soldiers, however, were not put under any scrutiny. This suggests a moralising discourse on prostitution, and the imbalance in attitudes between men vis-à-vis women suggests again that women's transgressions of the moral norms and the responsibility for these transgressions was not seen similarly to that of men.

The focus on the physical health of sex workers has led to a neglect of the social aspects of their lives. Little is known of these women beyond some limited aspects of their health, and a proper social analysis is needed in order to contextualise these findings, which would also contribute to more appropriate and effective policies in this field. The presumption that HIV transmissions occur through sexual contact forces us to challenge what we know about the sexual norms that restrict women's sexuality and their interaction with men in general, bringing the concepts of sexuality and gender to the fore. When *devadasis* and sex workers in HIV prevention 'speak', their words and writings enable us to see ruptures in the discourse of pure and chaste womanhood, which is central to the idea of femininity in India. The existing research, fails to understand the conceptual tensions here – when conservative ideals of sexuality and discourses of purity and chastity prevail, how are we to understand the existence of sex workers? In most existing accounts of sex work and HIV prevention, these crucial aspects of gender and sexuality are ignored in the search for epidemiology.

Discourses around women and sexuality in India

When I started my fieldwork, there was little to help me develop my understanding of sexuality and women in India. On the one hand, *sensuality* has been long been a part of the Hindu religion, culture, society and social order. 'India' had produced the *Kama Sutra*, which praises sexuality and sexual practices and devotes a whole chapter to courtesans and prostitution. Erotic temples with carvings of people in all sorts of gender combinations, in the most imaginative positions, are found all over India, such as in Konark in Orissa. On the other hand, in writings about women's behaviour, positions related to kinship and their functional role in the homes, women are associated with purity, family honour, spirituality, asexuality and domesticity.[2] Valuable as these writings are, they are restricted to practices around gender, and do not touch upon the issues of sexuality and sexual behaviour, particularly in reference to erotica.

Women's subordinate role in northern India, first under control of the father, then the husband and, finally, the son, has been explored by Jeffery (1979), Jeffery *et al.* (1989) and Jeffery and Jeffery (1996). Works by Caplan (1985), Hancock (1999), Jeffery (1979) and Trawick (1990) all set out an upper-class and upper-caste discourse regarding women. These authors discuss norms that restrict women's behaviour towards men, suggesting that women in India have little autonomy over the issues of reproduction and sexuality, such as who they marry and who they are expected to have sex with. Femininity is associated with purity, submissiveness and chastity, and modesty in dress, speech and behaviour. A practical method of monitoring women's honour is *purdah*, the seclusion of women from the public. Jeffery's study (1979) of a respected Muslim community in Delhi suggests that *purdah* is not just a Muslim practice but a ubiquitous South Asian practice that takes varying regional forms. Variations in *purdah* range from covering the body with a full *burkha* that has a net over the eyes, to covering the head with the sleeve of a *sari*, to covering the whole upper body with a *dupatta* (a scarf that is folded over the chest), to avoiding eye contact and communication with men completely.[3]

These ideas of women's honour and purity have been traced to colonial processes and also to the idea of women as the subjects of nationalist struggles for independence. The contemporary ideas that idolise women as mothers and as submissive runs parallel to Gandhian ideas about women that were put forward in the nationalist movement (see, for example, Chatterjee 1989; Dell 2005, Kishwar 1986; Patel 1988; and Tambiah 2005, who reported similar findings in Sri Lanka). Ideas about women as mothers, bringing up children and being inherently chaste, passive and non-violent (Kishwar 1986; Patel 1988) were discoursive tools in the negotiation of colonialism in the struggle for independence, and were used to show the moral superiority of the Indians over the British. Women's bodies acted as the symbols of the purity of their families, communities/castes and the nation at large (Chatterjee 1989). Women's purity maintained the purity of the race. The discourse of women as chaste and under *purdah* crystallises the idea of women's honour as family honour (although the degree of this varies locally). Women's honour as the symbol of family honour, inter-related with the reputation of their family members, communities and castes, explains how and why women's transgressions are judged more harshly: more is at stake (see Das 1975 for a discussion).

These norms are not always adhered to, however. They are challenged by the everyday practices of *devadasis* and sex workers, and by love marriages. These ruptures in normative sexual behaviour challenge the project of sexual purity, in that not all women act upon the norms of sexuality and some men seek sex outside their marriages. These sexual norms stand out as based on upper-caste and upper-class views, and not as universal and prescribed positionings.

Besides the dominant upper-caste discourse of women's sexuality, one that is restrained to marriage, other counter-hegemonic voices do exist on the margins. *Devadasis* set markers and represent disruptions to ideas about women as either controlled virgins or monogamous, auspicious wives. The institution of *devadasi* has been traced back to AD 100. Although the *devadasis* have received some recent attention, much of it has been historical in its focus (see, for example, Kersenboom-Story 1987; Orr 2000) and lacks any discussion of contemporary *devadasis*. Very little is known of the contemporary *devadasi* institution, but there is evidence that the institution has not disappeared entirely, but exists in parts of Karnataka (Blanchard *et al.* 2005; O'Neil *et al.* 2004) and is tolerated underground. Beginning in the late nineteenth century, social reformists lobbied against the institution of *devadasis*, and eventually it was officially banned in the 1950s. These reforms were part of the construction of the nationalist ideology of women as pure, sexless and chaste. The concept of *devadasi* posed a threat to discourse of the Indian nation as pure and morally superior compared to the British in the discursive process of nation-building. From a structuralist viewpoint, the *devadasi* were the polar opposite of the idea of the pure women enshrined in the nationalist discourse and were seen as sexually active and thus impure and disease-ridden. Even worse, they were women who, at times, held powerful positions in their communities, and who gained impressive properties. Kirsti Evans (1998) has argued that – due to a lack of understanding of their rituals and the social relationships involved – this viewpoint essentialised the institution of *devadasi* as sexual service and 'sexualised' the institution as prostitution. Sexualising the *devadasi* institution again suggests a moralising attitude to women's (sexual) power, which is perceived as uncontrolled and against the dominant upper-caste ideology regarding gender and sexual norms.

These moral ideas inform how sex workers are seen contemporarily. Sex workers do not adhere to the moral norms of chastity and monogamy, and, because of this, they are heavily stigmatised. Sex workers are seen as the main vectors of HIV, a view maintained by the statistic that eighty-five per cent of HIV infections are sex work related (NACO 2004: 14). The persistence in focusing on sex workers as key figures in HIV prevention echoes the need to construct an 'other' in the nationalist project. Gisselquist and Correa (2006) argue that HIV transmission has for more than two decades been mistakenly associated with heterosexual commercial sex. They triangulated various data and suggested that, contrary to the above reported statistic, the rate of HIV transmission by sex workers is actually two to twenty-seven per cent [*sic*] of transmissions, rather than eighty-five per cent as suggested by NACO (2004: 14). Gisselquist and Correa (2006: 741) argue that persisting in blaming sex workers is due to cultural moralising. In this project, prostitutes are juxtapositioned as the 'other', in contrast with the 'good women' at home (Ghosh 2004: 108–10).

Ideas about women's roles as restricted to familial functions, under intense scrutiny in terms of what options they have due to the preoccupation with family, honour and chastity, and conservative ideas about sexuality, shaped my own initial understanding of women's positions in India before going to do my fieldwork. There was a gap between the upper-caste and class norms, and the literature on *devadasi* and sex workers in HIV prevention. The literature on HIV implies that not all women are bound by the discourse of women as monogamous, auspicious, sexually modest and economically looked after by their fathers, husbands and sons. If the normative idea of monogamy and sexual restriction to marriage is not 'true' then what could the sex workers tell us about sexuality in a context where sex is a taboo? How do Tamil sex workers fit into these moral codes and practices, and how generalisable are discourses of femininity to the realities of many women's lives?

Tamil discourses of gender

If we question the universalist assumption of gender and sexuality, women in India, Tamil Nadu and Chennai unfold as a heterogeneous group. Assuming a pan-Indian account of gender and femininity is an essentialising error: the position of women is deeply inflected by their caste, religious and class backgrounds. For example, there are regional differences between northern and southern India. On a range of scales, Tamil Nadu is among the most developed regions in India (on par with Kerala). Specifically, variables that relate to women – such as women's literacy, and infant and maternal mortality – suggest that women are in a better position in Tamil Nadu than elsewhere in India. Other examples of this include the tradition of bride wealth rather than dowry, the celebration of girls' puberty, and a low performance of female infanticide, all of which are perceived to reflect respect towards women. Dyson and Moore (1983) and Sundari Ravindran (1999) have suggested that the more 'advanced' position of women in Tamil Nadu is due to higher autonomy. Dyson and Moore (1983) argue that this is related to the predominant kinship system in southern India, in which cross-cousins (a cousin who is the child either of one's mother's brother or one's father's sister) marry each other. Women married according to these rules stay within their natal family. Other arguments suggest that the local agriculture – especially where the staple crop is rice – is more labour inten-sive than growing wheat, as in north India (Dyson and Moore 1983; see also Das 1975). This has required women's participation in the labour force and, thus, these authors argue, women have a relevant and respected role in the economy, which has led to respect for women in other areas of social life.

Other ideas about women's advanced position in Tamil Nadu relate to the Self-Respect Movement in Tamil Nadu, headed by E. V. Ramas-wamy, who took a deliberate stance against upper-caste ideas about caste and gender. The Self-Respect Movement valorised 'Tamilness' against a pan-Indian experience, but also encouraged marriages of partnership, the equality of women, and participation of members of the lower caste in poli-tics. Anandhi (1998) argues that, in the Self-Respect Movement's emphasis on equality for women, women were encouraged to take control over their bodies by using contraceptives, and marriage was encouraged as an indi-vidual choice based on love, rather than an economic–familial expectation (Anandhi 2005; George 2003; Gorringe 2005). Such stands question the patriarchal roots of marriage and provide some bases for women to claim more autonomy. Penny Vera-Sanso (2006) argues, however, that, in Tamil nationalist politics in the 1940s, some of these more radical ideas of E. V. Ramaswamy were dropped. Instead, Tamil nationalists emphasised a 'Tamil identity', in which part of the ideology was to see women as chaste and pure mothers and to valorise men as providers and protectors. Ironically, the latter stance is not very different from the pan-Indian nationalist stance. These ideas – of women's purity and honour as indicative of family honour – allow for much more scrutiny and control of women's behaviour than that of men.

Besides geographical divisions in India, caste and class status affect the position that women have. Findings from Van Hollen (2003) in Chennai suggest variations among women in terms of class. Her studies of poor women with regard to reproductive practices showed that these women were not only able to go out of their homes, but also had to do so, as their work was needed to provide a minimal family income. Working women like this might have more autonomy compared with their upper-class counter-parts. Swaminathan (2004) also reported an increased sense of self-worth among women who worked outside the home. Gorringe (2005) discusses

Dalit women's autonomy in relation to *Dalit* anti-caste movements in Tamil Nadu and argues that, even although *Dalit* women are more autonomous than upper-caste women as their work allows access to the outside world, they end up having a double burden of paid work and housework rather than more say in crucial aspects of their lives. A similar critique was also suggested by Swaminathan (2004). The upper castes can afford to keep their women in the house, but this does not necessarily mean that women who have access to the outside world are empowered. Sundari Ravindran (1999) reminds us that women's positions relative to men are multifaceted. She argues that women in Chennai are more autonomous in the public domain in comparison with their northern counterparts, but that they remain under the control of men in issues relating to the domestic sphere, and they do not have a voice when it comes to matters of sexuality.

Concerns about women's sexuality tie into ideas of gender and autonomy. Tamil discourses of femininity also idolise motherhood and women's self-sacrifice. Women's structural roles are related to domesticity: looking after the children, supporting the husband, maintaining the home and preparing the food. In her study of orthodox Tamil Brahman women's domestic rituals, Hancock (1999) suggests that these practices are not merely menial tasks, but are seen as symbolic rituals that construct and contain feminine power, *shakti*, which demands respect towards Tamil Nadu women in general. Wadley and others (1980a) suggest that the 'Powers of Tamil Women' give them such respect. Wadley (1980b) suggests that *shakti* is seen in godlike terms to empower women with the ability to control life and death. *Shakti* is associated with self-sacrifice, chastity, morality and creation (which is particular to *married* women with children), and this power makes women auspicious (Egnor 1980; Hancock 1999; Reynolds 1980). Women's auspiciousness derives from 'pure' behaviour and marriage, but inherent in women's lives are also inauspicious phases, such as menstruation, childbirth and widowhood (Hancock 1999).[4] Because women can have almost supernatural powers, they are seen to need to be kept under the control of the men (Egnor 1980; Wadley 1980b). Uncontrolled women's sexuality and sexual behaviour could have drastic effects and might lead to loss of family honour.

Transgressions of these moral norms can lead to domestic violence, ostracism and even death. Domestic violence – often seen as a tool used by men to maintain power in their own homes – is common in south India despite these claims to more autonomy and respect than elsewhere in India (for Chennai, see Geetha 1998; Go *et al.* 2003; Subadra 1999; for Kerala, see Busby 2000). The threat of violence ensures that women are submissive to patriarchy in general. Penny Vera-Sanso (2006) argues that men are violent when women challenge the social order: talk back, fail to make agreeable food, challenge the in-laws or when they are seen to be out of control (for example, if women go to work outside the home). Arguing that domestic violence is related to men maintaining a powerful position over women suggests that the discourses surrounding gender subjectivities and the norms that control women's behaviour and sexuality are not disembodied, but can potentially have destructive and dangerous material results. As women have very little power over questions of sexuality and live on the brink of violence, it is not surprising that HIV infection is also prevalent in Tamil Nadu. The above arguments highlight that women's honour is tied to women's sexuality and sexual purity, and show how little space they have to manoeuvre within norms preserved by moral, physical and social sanctions.

Overall, very little academic literature exists regarding the sexuality of women with specific reference to sexual behaviour and erotic pleasure in India. The dominant ideas of sexuality relate to upper- and middle-class ideals. These upper-caste and class norms privilege keeping women at home, and women who work outside the home have been stigmatised as less 'chaste'. Women's work has been more prevalent in the south of India, particularly among poor, often lower-caste women, which has led to a discourse according to which women from these communities are less concerned about restricting their sexuality (Kishwar 1999: 216–21). However, being able to go to work does not mean that these women are immune to the norms of sexual restrictions and monogamy. Questions of sexuality cannot be essentialised to particular groups in this way but are complex and individually understood.

An example of individually negotiated sexuality comes from Viramma, a Scheduled Caste woman who told her life story to Racine and Racine (Viramma *et al.* 1997) and gave an account of her life that involved sexual desire and pleasure. Jyoti Puri (1999) talked about the restricted desires of middle-class women. These accounts suggest that there are times when individuals can recreate and challenge norms around sexuality, times when they may accept and enact them and others when they may subvert them. Even if Tamil women have access to work and are theoretically seen as more autonomous, they are still bound by the prevailing sexual norms. Sex workers are vulnerable to the discourses of HIV and patriarchal attitudes towards women, and these attitudes are also present in academic writings about sex workers in India, in which sex workers are seen as victims and/ or culprits.

Development approach on sex work

The rise of HIV in India and Tamil Nadu has brought a new interest in the sexual behaviour of people who are seen as risky to themselves and others. I classify some of this writing as the 'development approach to sex work,' by which I mean those (albeit rare) accounts that address social concerns to do with sex workers and their lives that emphasise empowerment and human rights. Nonetheless, I suggest, the aim of the development approach is still to minimise the risk of HIV, and so these writings also fail to depart from the viewpoint of HIV prevention.

Similar to the Western debate about sex work as oppression or profession, and sex workers as agents or not, attitudes toward sex workers in publications about sex work/HIV in India range from perceiving them as victims to seeing them as self-determined individuals. Many writings characterise sex workers as socially stigmatised, exploited, oppressed and powerless. Rao *et al.* (2003) go to the extent of arguing that the women even see themselves as fallen and outcaste. While this may be so, using this as evidence of victimhood is a one-sided interpretation of these women's agency, and it fails to understand that women might have differing reasons for describing themselves as 'fallen and outcaste'. By contrast, Oldenburg (1990) argues that the lifestyle of courtesans in Lucknow was actively chosen and reflected the women's desire for financial independence and freedom from sexual control, in order to overcome the restrictions on female behaviour and the attempts to limit women to domestic roles. Even so, women in such positions may choose not to 'flaunt' their independence to outsiders.

A victimising assumption that 'no woman would be a prostitute if they had a choice' is present (for example) in discussions by Pardasani (2005) and Rao *et al.* (2003). This assumption reflects the moralising ideas of upper-caste sexuality in its underlying idea that having sex with many men for money is exploitative as well as against dominant understandings of monogamy. Rao *et al.* (2003: 595, 600) argue, somewhat contradictorily, that women do sex work as the only alternative to destitution, given that sex work can provide twice the amount of money compared with the other jobs that are available to them. The assumption that is reflected here is that sex work is incomprehensible as a preferable option, even if it provides more money – it cannot be an active choice, but one that has to be explained as an act of desperation to be understandable. Similarly, Pardasani (2005) argues that women end up in sex work as a means to survive the economic conditions because of their ignorance. Her argument echoes the abolitionist stance to prostitution: that some women are unable to understand their best interests and fall into prostitution. These views ignore the agency of the women concerned and assume a universal mode of sexuality that corresponds to upper-caste ideals, and concludes that sex work is a matter of desperation and sex workers are victims.

Although some of this work essentialises sex workers as victims and without agency, the rise of the notion of sex as work has allowed space for identity-based politics. In some contexts HIV has – ironically – created a space within which sex workers can fight for their rights. Becoming empowered in this way is seen as crucial for effective HIV prevention in the development approach of sex-work literature (Asthana and Oostvogels 1996; Blanchard *et al.* 2005; Evans and Lambert 1997; Evans 1998; Gooptu 2000; Jayasree 2004; Nag 2001; O'Neil *et al.* 2004; Pardasani 2005; Rao *et al.* 2003). Ghosh (2004: 110) argues that sex workers in *Durbar Mahila Sangham*, the first sex workers' collective in Calcutta, actively shifted opinions away from the idea that sex workers are 'polluted' (*sic*), towards the language of human rights and particularly that of workers' rights. Despite this, however, the debate about the right to (sex) work (in safe conditions) is sparse in Indian sex-work theorisation.

One exception to this is Jayasree (2004), who takes a human rights approach to sex work and discusses the problems of sex workers in Kerala from the sex workers' point of view. This approach criticises the Indian legal system, which allows interpretation of the law against sex workers and condones acts of violence against sex workers by legal authorities such as the police. Jayasree also argues that sex work is 'work' and emphasises sex workers' right to oppression-free sexuality, separating sexuality from the act of selling sex. Another example is Amin (2004), who argues that HIV prevention cannot be a narrow health-focused approach to sex work, but must be an overall human rights-based approach that addresses advocacy, stigma and violence, and that targets people with power around sex workers, such as pimps, brokers, brothel owners, clients and partners (Amin 2004).

Conclusion

To a greater or lesser degree, all of the academic writings on sex work discussed in this chapter focus on HIV. Attempts to understand the experiences of the sex workers has moved a step closer to granting the sex workers agency rather than leaving them as 'objects' of HIV prevention – which sees them as victims or as scapegoats for the spread of HIV. However, research that calls for empowerment and human rights does not question the current state of affairs. Namely this approach neglects that fact that India and Tamil Nadu are highly patriarchal societies in which economic survival is increasingly difficult, poverty is strife, violence against women is common, and women do not have a say in matters of sexuality. Moreover, work which suggests that involving the sex workers is crucial to making HIV prevention more effective is still reduced conceptually to aspects of health. Overall, associating sex work with HIV fails to understand the social realities of the sex workers lives outside/beyond the discourse of HIV. Sex-working women's identities and experiences remain absent from these writings.

This provides the rationale for my research, which aims at bringing out the experiences of the sex workers. What are the major issues in their lives? What kind of experiences have they had while doing sex work? When the NGOs address sex workers as key actors in HIV prevention, what is the relationship between the sex workers and the NGOs? What kind of governance is created through this relationship? Is it poverty and being victims of male sexuality that motivates women to do sex work, or are there agentic, empowered or unconventional choices behind this? Can sex workers have power in the sex-work encounter when women in general do not have power in relation to sex? How do they feel about sex work against the backdrop of strict chastity norms? What was the meaning of sexuality in their lives? Can sex workers say something about sexuality outside the dominant discourse? Clearly, there are things unsaid and unwritten in the dominant discourse on sexuality that the HIV prevention discourse does not explain. Sex workers and their own perspectives on their lives are key to exploring such questions.

3   Women in sex work

Over my year in Chennai, I interviewed fifty-six women for this book and one of the topics that was discussed in the interview was how and why they had started to sell sex. This chapter uses this interview data to broaden current representations of sex workers (beyond seeing only their roles in HIV prevention) and to emphasise the socially complex realities and multiplicity of other social aspects of the lives of the sex workers. As Nandini Gooptu (2000) found in her research within the Calcutta Sonagachi red light district, sex workers are a heterogeneous group. Despite their differences, however, sex workers in Calcutta deployed simplistic representations of themselves as a strategic act: HIV provided an issue around which sex workers were able to mobilise. HIV can act as a common enemy, which provides the sex workers with a degree of unity that otherwise they find hard to achieve. Such a strategy has not been successful in Chennai: women have not mobilised in these ways, and in answering the question 'why not?' my findings highlight how 'flat' a health-focused representation of HIV is. It neither takes women's heterogeneity into account nor addresses the social problems behind the risk of HIV. Sex work in not restricted to HIV nor experienced in isolation from the other roles that women have, and these other roles contextualise why they engage in sex work. Therefore, although sex work was the primary focus of the interviews with the women, the discussions ranged over aspects of women's other identities as well.

It is hard to approach sex workers in Chennai without engaging with the HIV 'industry' in some degree. There is no red light district in Chennai. For someone who does not know the deviant spaces of Chennai, the most obvious context where one can make contact with the women is through NGOs that are engaged in HIV prevention work. Therefore, to begin with I spent time in the offices of the NGOs, and met the women who came in for meetings, either as peer educators or as members of the 'target group' – women who were by default described as sex workers. As they got to know me better they invited me to join their lives outwith the NGOs. I began to visit a number of women's homes on a regular basis and then to conduct interviews, either at their homes or in the NGO premises. I wanted to avoid the 'survey-like' approach deployed by the NGOs when they collected information, not only to differentiate myself from the approaches of the NGO staff, but also to avoid categorising the women before letting them explain themselves.

My intention throughout was to allow the women to talk about themselves in ways in which they found meaningful and relevant, and in large measure I think I was successful. In the analysis below I have tried to maintain the complexity and ambiguities that emerged as women talked about their lives. For some women, I did not have the opportunity to return to them and fill in gaps – for example in the basic demographic data. Not all women were as forthcoming as the eighteen who were my key informants. For these eighteen, in addition to several somewhat formal interviews each, I also met them regularly much more informally. In these varied discussions the women talked about their families, women's gender position, sexuality, the NGOs, violence against sex workers and why they got into sex work. This approach allowed the multiple roles and dimensions of these women's identities to emerge.

This chapter describes the women's identities with reference to age, education, number of children, cohabitation, sexual orientation and sexual partners. It also analyses the reasons the women gave for entering sex work. Four in-depth accounts start the chapter, so that women's own voices set the scene. These accounts show how multiple roles and the contingencies of individual histories come together in the lives of individual women, and (crucially) how the women themselves make sense of these patterns: how they are able to find coherence in their own narratives. In conjunction, the findings introduced in this chapter lay the foundation of the range of topics that will be analysed in later chapters on the NGOs (Chapter 4), problems encountered in sex work and negotiating these problems (Chapter 5), and gender and sexuality (Chapter 6).

Mercy, Zaima, Uma and Kuntala

The four individual narratives from these women provide a somewhat linear sense of how different events occurred in these women's lives. These accounts should not be generalised to all sex workers, nor even to the all the women who were interviewed; rather, they should be seen as illustrative of the different experiences of the four women. They are (among other things) gendered, sexual, emotional and social beings within specific social contexts. Their lives led to sex work in different ways, and they felt differently about it. These accounts draw on between two and four formal interviews for each of the four women, as well as on several informal chats. In most cases, these interviews were recorded; in the few cases in which they were not, I made notes as soon as possible. The interviews were conducted with a research assistant, and sometimes the women had a female friend present, who was also a sex worker. These accounts are often not focused on the particular, as is the autobiography of Viramma, a Tamil *Dalit* woman whose whole life story was recorded (Viramma *et al.* 1997). Rather, they are products of the interviews that we had, with my particular interests in sex work, gender and sexuality, and the women's knowledge of this. In the interviews, these women reflected on their experiences as young women, talked about marriage and how they got into sex work, and shared their views on gender, sex work, men, sex, and the issues that sex workers are collectively facing. Some of what they said shows quite neatly the networks that exist amongst the women, and the accounts suggest some similarities, but also show differences in their interpretations of their situations.

The reasons the women gave for entering sex work were told with hindsight and in particular contexts. What they saw as the reasons why and how they entered sex work might have changed overtime, and they might have talked about them differently depending on whom they were talking to. Because of the stigmatised nature of sex work in the Indian context, it seems likely that these women felt the need to justify why they do what they do, which might lead to an inclination to represent themselves as victims acting in desperate circumstances. We must keep in mind that the women might have told me their accounts as intentional positionings rather than reflecting the past events 'truthfully'. Their freedom to choose how to represent themselves is part of the agency that they had. By trying to convince me with politically correct accounts of victimisation, they might have also been trying to avoid further questions, or potentially, to protect themselves and their reputation. I do not want to dismiss the experiences of the women as simply 'stories', excuses or appeals to gain my sympathy and suggest that their accounts have no experiential basis, but nor do I want always to accept them as straightforward factual accounts of 'what happened'. Each account is a blend of memories, justifications, reflections and creation. In another time and place, with a different interlocutor and audience, the combination may have led to narratives that were different in detail but not, I think, in overall orientation.

Mercy

When I met Mercy in one of the NGOs for the first time, she was very pregnant and glowing. She was a 25-year-old Malayali (from Kerala, the state neighbouring Tamil Nadu in south India), who had studied up to the ninth standard at school, undertaken a beautician course, migrated between Kerala and Gujarat, worked on a shrimp farm, and finally settled with her husband in Chennai. She had an arranged marriage when she was 17, and gave birth to a son. Her husband was from Chennai. While she and her husband worked on the shrimp farm in Gujarat, she had an affair with another woman.

> There was trouble between Saheli [another woman] and her husband. As she was always around he suspected a relationship between the pair of us. So as it became such a big problem I decided to come to Madras with my husband ...
>
> > (Interview transcript: p. 1, line 42; p. 2, line 2, 2 June 2005)

Mercy: My husband had a job as a security guard here in Madras for the Hindustan Engineering College. We were happy together, he was earning well and I stayed at home, he wouldn't send me anywhere. We were comfortable and jolly. Then on his way to work he died in an accident. It was about a year after the wedding. My son was 1 year old when he died. I've only one son.

Salla/translator: So, did you return to your mum's or your mother-in-law's?

Mercy: Me and my mother-in-law never got on so I stayed here alone with my son. My Mum and Dad were a help to me. But I decided I would stay alone. I knew how to be a beautician. (When) I had finished my studies and was a year at home I did a 6 months' course in it. So I told my mum I would manage and set up or work in a beauty parlour. She said, 'the choice is yours; if you stay at home you don't seem able to cope.' So I spent 6 months at home after his death, that was all, then I left my son with my mum and promised I'd give her money monthly. I got work at the beauty parlour and it was going fine when suddenly I got underpaid. I said, 'this isn't enough', I got Rs. 1,250 a month. Well, so I thought, 'I don't need this.' So I knew a broker/agent for make-up and I went to him and told him my work situation. He said there was a man, some manager who would give me work if I 'went' with him. He openly told me. I was scared and was put off, but the broker said, 'once you're in you get a good salary, and it is only for one day, not even that, you only have to go with him once.' I thought about it hard, I couldn't be alone without any money, so I finally accepted it. I 'went' with him once and he gave me Rs. 1,800 and promised to find me work. And right the next day he phoned and said someone needs a beautician. I went and was working for X [a famous film actress who's old and is still acting]. I was working there for 4 months, living in as well.

(Interview transcript: p. 1, lines 8–30, 18 February 2005)

While working there, Mercy met a girl, Latika:

The pair of us got to be really close. So 6–7 months went by. You know 'lesbian'? Well, me and Latika got into that. Actually since when I was young I had these desires. I don't know how I got married. I never desired to be with a man. Even now it's the same. I see sex (work) as a job; I can't show my preference in that. So I was there a year and we were so close.

(Interview transcript: p. 2, lines 3–6, 18 February 2005)

After persuading her parents, Latika moved in with Mercy so that neither of them would have to live alone, but they did not tell anyone about the fact that they were a couple. Latika was looking after Mercy's son and Mercy was earning money.

I've actually tied a *thali* to her. I took her to a Hindu temple, because actually both Latika and I are Hindu. My husband was Christian which is how I got the name Mercy, so I call myself, Sathia-Mercy as my Hindu name is Sathia. So at this temple we exchanged rings and I tied a *thali* onto her. And as close as we were, her mum came and gave us hassle. Latika didn't show her *thali* out publicly, she wore it on a chain.

(Interview transcript: p. 2, line 45; p. 3, line 4, 2 June 2005)

Trouble started when Latika's parents wanted to marry her off but she refused. Latika attempted suicide when she was pressured to leave Mercy, but eventually consented and went back to her parents' house, where Mercy visited her:

Latika's mum said, 'Please don't come to see Latika any more. Stay some days without seeing her. If you want speak to each other do it on the phone.' Even if we speak on the phone she [Latika] won't let me be, she'll cry and cry so much that the man at the telephone booth asks me what's up and tells me to get her whatever she's crying for! So I said, 'With this I'll end it. I shan't phone either, forget me. I'll not come to your area.' Latika didn't know what her mum had said to me and I didn't tell her so Latika was asking me 'Why, for what reason?' I said, 'Get married to someone and live with them, and you live your life and I mine.' And she asked me if that's what the friendship was worth. I said it had nothing to do with the friendship. I told her to get married and be happy and well and promised I'd visit her wherever she was as a friend. And she said, 'I don't care if I die, I don't want to get married.' Well, so that problem finished. Then suddenly a call came 'I can't stay here, take me away somewhere. They tell me that I'm this old and I'm still not married', Latika was sobbing. Latika's Mum works as a housemaid in Madras [Chennai] so I went over to where she works and asked her why she was scolding Latika like that. I explained that I'd had Latika in tears to me on the phone. The mum replied coldly and sort of told me to mind my own business. 'You don't have to ask me that', she said, 'don't meddle in this'. So I left. And Latika phoned again that day and said 'Please don't take this as me scolding you but I'm asking you not to phone me again or visit.' I had a cell phone and I wanted to smash it I was so angry. It was because I had the phone that she could phone me so I threw it and it broke into pieces. I left it and she wandered around from a long time without my number unable to speak with me. Suddenly one day around 8 pm at night she was there standing at the door. I was amazed. I thought she must have come with her mum but she'd come alone with her suitcase. When I asked here what happened, she said her mum had quarrelled a lot and said 'You phone that Mercy up all the time and chat away moaning. If you want to go, go, but I'll have nothing more to do with you, you can forget me.'

(Interview transcript: p. 6, line 29;
p. 7 line 10, 18 February 2005)

So, Latika ran back to Mercy because her family still wanted to marry her off and because they questioned her about Mercy and their relationship. At this point, Latika's parents came looking for her and, when Mercy and Latika moved, her parents thought that Mercy had trafficked her. When they found Mercy and Latika, they beat Mercy up. Mercy filed a case against them. In the end, Latika moved back to her family, although she calls Mercy once a month, and Mercy lives alone with her son. After Latika, she has not had any long-term relationships. In the future, she would like to live with her son, but maybe to have a wife also.

Mercy identifies herself as a lesbian, an unusual and rare public identity in India. It is not unusual in the West to have sex workers who are lesbians, but in India, lesbianism is rare or, at least, not discussed.

There must be countless women like me who are keeping it inside their heart and suffering. I often wonder if a man likes a woman and goes to take her on how would it be? In my heart I am a man because I'm a lesbian. My outward appearance is female but in my heart I am a man. I think 'I am like this, I'll keep my girl like this', that's what I think. But, having said that, I don't go around harassing people! I want to keep a lady as a wife. Just like how a man desires to keep his wife, those sorts of desires I get as well. It is all a dream ...

(Interview transcript: p. 6, lines 17–24, 2 June 2005)

I see it as purely different from my work. You know Nagalakshmi at the office? Well, he said when he found out I was lesbian that there was a lot of work for me in Bangalore where lesbian girls were in demand. The job was lucrative but I didn't like the idea. I like to go with those I like. I take sex work just as a job, I don't have a pleasure from it. I don't want to go doing it for other women.

(Interview transcript: p. 3, lines 3–13, 2 June 2005)

Mercy provides a powerful statement of her agency in how she defines her work and how she describes the way in which she regulates her desire, separating these two aspects. She goes on to describe herself as a man instead of a woman; she says she prefers to wear trousers and T-shirts, and that she also has manly characteristics, such as being bold and aggressive and protective over women around her. She talks about the NGOs and says that they are generally good and that what they give is important. She is not very critical of them, and only when I asked her about lesbians' rights did she agree that that would be an important form of action.

When Mercy and Latika lived together, at work Mercy witnessed her boss 'lying in a strange way' with a man who was not her husband. Mercy was shocked and quit working for her as a beautician. She used her contacts to get jobs in the film industry. After a while, however, the shootings did not provide enough money and Mercy got into sex work for the second time. She understood that these relationships were part of the film industry and, although she did not like the idea, she understood that it might happen to her again. So when Zaima, her friend, who was also a sex worker and a pimp, and who worked in the film industry, called up a man, she knew what was expected from her: 'I got home and started thinking: I'm not going to have another marriage and I can't sustain my body on mud so I'll have to do what humans do' (interview transcript: p. 8, lines 43–5, 18 February 2005). We talked about sexual acts with clients. She said it is all play on her part when she is with clients. She would only touch their head and talk to them nice because otherwise, she says, they would not come back to her. She was embarrassed when saying that she would not give anything else except what is 'normal', but she will let them touch her or take her clothes off if they pay for it. She has six regular clients whom she meets about twice a month. When I first met her, she was pregnant by a client. She did not want the baby and looked for an abortion, but the pregnancy was too far advanced. However, she grew attached to the idea of another child, and in the end was disappointed when it was stillborn.

Zaima

I met Zaima in one of the HIV prevention NGOs. She worked as a field-worker in an NGO and later started to work as a counsellor because she had a lot of contacts and she was known to work well. She was about 50 at the time of study, and lived in the suburbs of Chennai with her husband, two sons and daughter-in-law. Zaima was often in a good mood and ready to crack jokes and have a laugh, but at the same time there was something broken and melancholic about her.

She was born to a very poor family. Her mother was a sex worker, although Zaima understood this only much later. Once, her mother had a partner who set his eyes on Zaima and he coerced her into have sex with him. At this time, Zaima was 13. 'That time', Zaima says, 'I did not know anything about sex or anything wrong with that' (interview transcript: p. 1, lines 4–5, 9 February 2005). Soon after, because the family did not have much money, her mother sent her to live with another client. At the age of 15, Zaima had her first periods and, she said, she had also gained some sense and refused to do sex work anymore.

At this point in her life, some neighbours intervened and sent her to work as a helper in a 'decent' family. Once, when she was shopping for the family, a man 'put his eye' on her. They became friends, and they met some-times. However, the family found out about this and called Zaima's mother. They refused to tolerate this inauspicious behaviour and they asked Zaima's mother to collect her. The man, however, married Zaima and they lived happily together. He worked as a TV mechanic and earned good money, although they did not save any of it: instead, they went to the cinema, ate in hotels, etc., enjoying themselves. Zaima is a Muslim and at this time she used to wear a *burkha* when they went out. She said this had been a good time in her life.

But then, her mother's partner gave her a hard time. Once, when they were alone, he tried to have sex with her and said she should marry him. She rejected this, saying: 'You are my mother's partner; I'm married and a good woman now' (interview transcript: p. 1, lines 19–20, 9 February 2005). She felt that he was like a father to her and that he was, after all, a good man. She had a fight with her mother. She felt horrible the whole day and cried a lot. When her husband came home, he asked what was wrong but she complained she had body pains and that she was not feeling well. She cried all night. In the morning, he asked again and she decided to tell him what had happened, telling him her whole story. Instead of being understanding, he became suspicious. They started to have fights continuously; he questioned her doings, thinking she was flirting with other men, doing sex work, etc. Finally, she became so tense that she attempted suicide by taking poison. A neighbour rescued her and she recovered. The next time she tried to hang herself. She piled up boxes because the roof was so high and, while climbing up, they all fell and neighbours heard and rushed in (Zaima was laughing while telling me this.) The neighbours told her to leave the area because they were worried about the trouble that a suicide would cause for them, and they beat her. Zaima was forced to go back to her mother's house. She tried to get her husband to take her back and she visited him but he had fixed in his mind that she was a bad, loose woman and he told her to find one of her clients as a new husband. She was about 17 years old at this point.

Having been back at her mother's house for about 2–3 months, her mother's partner approached her again, offering to marry her. At this point, she felt she had no choice and accepted. They got married and she had a son. The husband was a business man and sold lorries. He was away for months and then brought a folder of money for Zaima to buy household goods. They lived together for 5 years. Then she started bleeding from her *loop* (IUD) and removed it. Because of this, she got pregnant again and had another son. Her husband started to give her trouble again, demanding to have sex with Zaima's mother. She tried to persuade them to have sex outside her home, so she would not get a bad reputation. Next, her husband demanded to have sex with both of them together. Zaima felt she had no choice and so they did. Eventually, she said it was not good and asked her mother to move out (Zaima dried her eyes silently while telling me this). Despite their differences, Zaima was very attached to her mother and she grieved deeply for her when she died during my fieldwork.

Zaima's landlady, who was a broker, had followed carefully what happened and suggested clients to her when she saw that she needed money. The landlady's son also wanted Zaima and so she had sex with him, thinking she could get her own house like this. He did not give anything, though, and she says she felt cheated. Somehow, Zaima managed to purchase a piece of land in an area of Chennai that was at the time merely on a dirt track. She built a thatched hut and still lives there; it was dark and very cramped. She still lives together with her husband. She says she dislikes being with him and he drinks and abuses her; she feels that he is the person who has 'spoilt' her life, but he is the father of her children. Her younger son is physically and mentally challenged, and she feels responsible for (and looks after) him.

Zaima started to work in the film industry as a make-up girl soon after her first husband left her. She said that the actors requested sex from her and other girls who worked there and that, slowly, she got into the profession of sex work. She told me she was very beautiful when she was young – and she still is – and that she had a lot of clients, but she did not save any of the money. Now she is too old to work and she longs for peace in her life. She lives on the small salary she gets from the NGO and pimping younger sex workers.

> Nowadays, I'm not doing sex work and even if I don't feel like doing it, when I'm tempted to do it I pray to God to somehow cancel it. One part of my heart says that if I go I will get at least some Rs. 500 and I'll even fix the appointment but another part of me prays to the God to somehow cancel it.
>
> (Interview transcript: p. 2, lines 37–41, 9 February 2005)

She is very bitter about her life and experiences; she recalls being raped and she feels that she was cheated at whatever she did. Her husband and her oldest son abuse her verbally. The only things she cites as pleasurable and meaningful in her life are her counselling work, which serves a means of being able to eat, the Islamic traditions that she likes, and occasional lesbian encounters with her friends. Her relationship to other women is striking and unusual.

Zaima: That [relationships with women] is for fun and I will do it rarely and it will be with close friends. Now here they talk about Komala and me and we both attended a *party* [a client] and it happened then, but it's not a habit. I had another friend who had the same name as myself and both of us were drunk. And that happened because of my husband when he came to know that I was a sex worker and then he started blackmailing me saying that 'You are mine and you have to pleasure me, so bring one of your friends and let me be with her. See I'm not going to be with her lifelong, it's just for fun.' I thought, 'OK if I satisfy him maybe he will take care of me.' So I introduced one friend, she was also from a poor family and she was a CSW [commercial sex worker]. He asked us to have sex and we did it for him but I enjoyed it and so that is in the corner of my mind always. So now with Komala, I just have fun and we tease each other and to Komala I say, 'Hey, you are my wife.' I don't do this as regular and it is just for fun and there is no shame in this because it is just for fun.

Bhavaani*: You said that you were with your husband and a friend as three persons. Even that habit was started by that man.

Zaima: . Yes, and even that habit was started by this man ... In the similar way I have introduced a lot of women to him and I will give Rs.50 or 100 to these women. What to do, I have told this man the truth and I also think about my handicapped son. Because of this weakness I used to give him a lot of leeway. I told you that he has always used me as a sacrificial sheep but this lesbian habit is just for fun, there are some who have this habit but I don't do it always.

(Interview transcript: p. 8, line 31;
p. 9, line 11, 9 February 2005)

Uma

I first met Uma, a young woman who smiled a lot, in one of Chennai's HIV prevention organisations, where she sat quietly. I met her the next time when I was doing social marketing of condoms with Lalitha, one of the fieldworkers. Uma told me she had malaria. We went to the tiny flat where she lived with her husband and son, and she seemed quite excited about me being there. During my fieldwork, her family moved due to family problems. Both of these typical slum flats were in poor areas in the north of Chennai. The second flat consisted of a room in a concrete two-floor building. The room was about 3 metres × 3 metres in size and had no bed, but had sleeping mats rolled up and standing in the corner, a small cooker under a tiny window, and a few pots and pans. They had a small cupboard that held their clothes and belongings. The fan on the roof went on and off because of electric cuts.

Uma is 25 years old and belongs to the *Naicker* caste (a higher caste of Telegu origin who have moved to Tamil Nadu). She studied up to the third grade and then helped her mother in selling fruits. She does not know how to read or write. She had a love marriage when she was 20 years old. Uma and her husband are from different backgrounds ethnically (he is Telegu, she is Tamil), in terms of class (his family lived in a rented house and hers in an owned house), and religiously (she is Hindu, he is a Christian), and, because of this, Uma's family does not approve of the marriage. The couple were in love for 3 years before they got married. 'What was your relationship like?' I asked. Uma explained that they exchanged letters, looks and the like; I asked if they were intimate and Uma blushed and laughed: '*Che ayaiyo*, dearie me, I did not know all that!' (interview transcript: p. 4 line

*Research assistant

32, 11 June 2005). Uma's father used to beat her for seeing him; everybody knew they were courting.

After her marriage, she gave birth to five children, four of whom died soon after birth. She felt that, at the hospital, they could not do anything to help her and the babies. She said the doctors wanted to keep the son who survived for monitoring, but she refused and blackmailed them to let her take the child home with her – she felt that experts had failed to look after her four other children and would probably fail with this son as well. She calls the boy 'the God's child' because he was born on Christmas Day. She is very happy about this son, although she was devastated when the other children died. Consecutive pregnancies have made her very weak, and Uma is very thin. After her last child was born, she went through the family planning operation (sterilisation), with the agreement of her husband and mother-in-law.

Before I met Uma, she had met another man, who keeps calling her and wants to marry her. He is a truck driver with a lot of money. He has given Uma a mobile phone, paid for her son's clothes, and given her money for rent. Uma says that she met the man as a client. Now they are in love and have been to the Marina beach, a common destination for newly-wed couples. It is obvious that Uma is very smitten with the man, and that she is not just meeting him for his money. However, Uma's husband found out about the affair, which resulted in a huge quarrel.

> My husband doesn't go to work. There is not even milk for the baby. That's why I started doing this. I suffered a lot, at that time; this man [the lover] was some help to me. He bought me milk and this and that. Everything. He gave me house rent. So like that it grew. What my husband said at the [police] station to him was: 'I married my wife through love marriage. You've only just come along.' The police beat him [the lover] up, with a stick. He [the husband] gave money [to the police] and made him be hit badly. The man said, 'I'll still speak [with her] however much I get beaten.' His [Uma's lover's] mother tells him not to speak with me, and she even tried committing suicide. She's told him he should marry the girl of her choice. He went and saw her, but he said he didn't want to marry her. They are also comfortably off. In one day he earns Rs. 2,000. He gets a monthly salary on top of that, and also any petrol or diesel which is left after he has delivered the tank, he sells on to other shops. In the petrol shops their books will be straight because they've received what they asked for. Then he sells the excess and makes Rs. 50,000.

> (Interview transcript: p. 5, lines 6–22, 11 June 2005)

When her husband found out about the affair, he beat her up, and she was also threatened by her natal family and her in-laws not to meet him again. In despair, Uma poured kerosene on herself, wanting to die. She suffered minor burns on her stomach and chest and had to spend a week in the hospital. She decided to stay with her husband because she did not want to lose her son. She said she feels sorry that her husband, who used to be a good man, has now started to drink and mentally abuse her: 'Have you been to the brothel again, have you met your boyfriend again?' (field notes: 10 March 2005). She feels guilty for what happened and she understands that there is more at risk than just her own feelings because her sister and mother have threatened to kill themselves if she continues to meet her lover. After further discussion about what she wants herself, she started to cry and said she would like to talk to her boyfriend.

Regarding sex work, Uma told me that she works on a full-time basis and that her clients are generally autorikshaw drivers and businessmen. She earns Rs. 300–1,000 per client, and she usually has three clients per day. She said she will 'give anything' because she needs the money. If she complains, her pimp will say: 'Why are you complaining, you got the money, you have been paid' (field notes: 10 March 2005). Uma argues that men will come (to sex workers) because their wives will not do impure things. She often works with Payal, her best friend, and recalled moments when they were asked to have sex together with a man:

> [Sometimes] he'll [the client] want us both there, for company. And by company he means we are naked and stroke him and that, whilst the other has sex.
> (Interview transcript: p. 6, lines 21–2, 11 June 2005)

Salla: Where do you usually go?
Uma: We go to houses. If someone from the house has gone out, we'll go to lodges.[1]
> (Interview transcript: p. 7, lines 6–7, 11 June 2005)

I asked if she and Payal ever met 'nice clients' (in contrast with the violent or cold men that they described). In this particular interview Uma and Payal were there together, and their initial answer was that, yes, some clients are rich and give a lot of money, mobile phones, *saris*, etc. Then they said, rather vaguely, that some are gentle, and that they will adjust to whatever the men want. Uma says that if they (sex workers) are harsh on the men, the men will take them by force – so if the women are nice to them, the men will also treat the women with care. But she also recalled a recent incident when ten men gang-raped her: only one man used a condom.

Kuntala

I met Kuntala for the first time in one of the peer educator's annual meetings. She was very beautiful and slim, spoke very well and I was impressed by how articulate she was. She was always very honest and frank. She welcomed me and my research assistant very warmly every time we went to see her, and she said she was always very relieved after talking with us. Kuntala lived with her husband and two children, 8 and 7 years old, in a thatched-roof hut that belonged to her father. They had a bed, a small cooking space, a cupboard and a small black-and-white TV. She has also adopted her nephew, who is around 15. Her other sister lives nearby.

Kuntala comes from a family of four children. Her father was a farmer and they had their children well educated. One sister became a nurse and another earned a BSc degree. However, one of the sisters had mental health problems and committed suicide. Kuntala says that, because of this, her mother is now also mentally affected and has been admitted to a local mental health hospital. Her mother, otherwise, wandered around the streets pointlessly. Bhavaani, my research assistant and I met her mother once: her dress was old and dirty and her hair stood up. Despite this, when she spoke to Bhavaani she was quite collected and talked to her in Telegu, asking about her caste and background.

Kuntala completed school up to the tenth standard. She was married off when she was 15 because her family had problems; she said her parents thought that at least one of the children should be settled. She said she was totally ignorant about marriage and felt as if she was still a child. She recalled that she did not even have time to have a 'good time' with her husband because she became pregnant immediately and had two children. She said she did not know how to look after the children, had no interest in being a mother and that she would push her baby away when it was crying. Her children were brought up by her sisters and mother. She did not want her second child, but the pregnancy was too far to terminate. Against her family members' will she went through sterilisation after her second child, threatening to go to the police if they tried to stop her. She was lonely and jealous of her peers, who were still going to school and college. Kuntala says that, at the time, she longed for company and started to go out more and, in this way, came to sex work:

> I didn't have anybody to talk to about my husband and problems. Both my sisters were like that, asocial or mental. I was social but there was no company, I was unable to be myself or free. When I tried to look for company from outside, other people pulled me into this [sex work]. I needed support and companionship but they turned out bad.
>
> (Interview transcript: p. 3, lines 37–40, 11 May 2005)

Aged 24, Kuntala said she enjoyed being a mother and liked being with her children, wanting to raise them well and make them smart and not easily deceived. She also wanted to make sure her children trusted her with all their worries. Especially, she said she wanted to empower her daughter. Her children were studying in English to make sure they get good opportunities in life. She was proud of her children and it seemed like she had adopted motherhood as her identity, rather than using it to explain her sex work.

At one point Kuntala worked for an international aid organisation as a cleaner, but her travelling expenses were so high that she spent her entire salary on that. By the time of my fieldwork she had stopped working as a sex worker, as her husband told her to stay at home – the work in the organisation also served as a pretext for getting out of the house – despite the fact that her children's school fees had not been paid. She raised heartfelt concerns about being exposed as a sex worker:

> Whenever I do sex work, I'm worried about other people. I think if anybody has seen me, I have no peace of mind. After I have stopped I feel better, I feel free, strong. If they give any job, I will go.
>
> (Interview transcript: p. 2, lines 17–20, 4 March 2005)

Kuntala would like to get a proper job in the nearby area. She was very worried that her husband might find out about her sex work and she has stopped even being seen with other sex workers. She had already been beaten for going out, and said she would expect a much more violent reaction if her husband were to find out that she did sex work. He is an autorikshaw driver and is normally of good nature, but he drinks quite a lot and when he gets drunk, he becomes abusive and beats her.

> He always fights with me and then I think: 'I don't want to live with him.' I want to leave him. But then I think of my family and if I would leave people would blame me and think of me in bad name: she did all that … I'm always crying. Sleep is not coming. You are continuously doing like this, it becomes a problem. I'm worried about my family. I still have a brother who didn't get married. My older sister is not married because she is mental. Second sister became mental and died. After my father died, I'm the only one who is looking after the family. I am thinking about the family situation so I am unable to sleep. Every time after we fight, I think how I can leave but then I think what would happen to the others.
>
> (Interview transcript: p. 1, lines 26–9;
> p. 2, 21–7, 4 March 2005)

If the people from the neighbourhood or her relatives speak badly about her, her husband becomes angry, drinks and abuses her. 'I tell him off when he's sober and then he says he's so sorry. He does not apologise but says he will not scold her again' (interview transcript: p. 1, lines 6–9, 11 May 2005). He is suspicious when Kuntala goes out with other women from HIV-awareness NGOs because these women openly say that they are sex workers. For that reason, she no longer dares to talk to them.

> I don't go often [to meetings] because I'm afraid that he will find out and I know that if he will understand what is going on, my family will be affected, my family's honour will be lost. The women in the area they make themselves public. It's fine if you talk in a meeting but even if you are with them in a bus they will come out as CSWs [commercial sex workers]. The way they talk, the way they tease each other, everybody will come to know. I'm scared to be seen with them. I never take the same bus, I don't want to be associated with them. I don't like it, I'm ashamed by it. When I go [to a meeting], I give an excuse where I'm going. But because my husband is an autorikshaw driver, he knows what kind of women they are. He knows what's going on around and so when I'm going to a meeting, he doubts me. That might be the reason why he gets drunk and scolds me. For the past 8 months I have completely stopped it. If I want pleasure, I can go to him. If something happens to me, who will look after the family? What I want is to eat, a dress and to be happy. What he earns is not enough for us and we have to get a loan. So for that reason I want to get another job.
> (Interview transcript: p. 3, lines 19–34, 11 May 2005)

While Kuntala was still in sex work, she was a home-based sex worker, using madams to find clients for her. She would get Rs. 200 per client, of which the madam took Rs. 100 as commission. She feels bad for having done sex work and she is worried about if anyone she knows has seen her. She has no peace of mind because of this and with all the family problems. Although she had done sex work, she hated it and despised herself for it. She said that, after she stopped doing sex work, she felt better, free and strong. I asked her if there was any difference in the intimacy between her and the clients and her husband, and she said that there was not much difference:

Kuntala: If he had been alright, if he had been very nice to me, I would have been here and I wouldn't have to go out. So there was not much difference. I thought there would have been something for me, but my husband simply drank all the money and the money I got from sex work was for my needs. I earned a bit for myself also.

Salla: What about the physical intimacy?
Kuntala: I was very simple with my clients. At least with my husband I
           think he is my husband and there is some emotional connection
           also. With the clients it was like a dead person.
                    (Interview transcript: p. 4, lines 1–8, 11 May 2005)

Heterogeneous group of women

Like this sample of four accounts, the women that were interviewed are
a heterogeneous group. Caste is generally a major distinguishing factor
in Tamil society; it can be seen in caste-divided party politics (Gorringe
2005), and in deep-rooted norms and practices (especially marriage) that do
not necessarily relate to the (Hindu) ideology of purity or religion (Deliege
1992; Trawick 1990). There are stereotypes that lower-caste women are less
observant of moral codes regarding sexuality. But the women I interviewed
came from all kinds of backgrounds. They said that they tend to know
which caste people in their neighbourhoods belong to but that it was not
important to them. For my informants, the meaning of caste had lessened,
perhaps because they all lived in poor urban areas that were mixed-caste,
mixed-religious settlements, similar to those that Vera-Sanso (2006)
described in Chennai, rather than areas dominated by certain castes as Gorringe (2006) found in Madurai. Caste was dismissed by my informants as
unimportant specifically because of the nature of sex work. In the words of
one of my informants: 'If we think about caste we will not get clients and if
they think of caste they will not get sex' (field notes: 22 December 2004).
Caste boundaries are often marked and maintained by women's purity and
chastity, and are tied up with reproduction within the caste, but these norms
and practices have to be suspended during sex work. Caste was not often
talked about beyond this. Some sex workers in Calcutta define themselves
as 'outcaste' (Rao *et al.* 2003) but not the women I met in Chennai. Most
women did not disclose their caste background, but the existence of some
women from higher castes, suggests that (low) caste was not a determining
factor among those that made women vulnerable to sex work.

The ethnic plurality of the population of Chennai and the fact that
Chennai is a target for migration were also represented in these women's
backgrounds. They were predominantly Tamil, but some were also from
neighbouring states: four from Andhra Pradesh (with Telegu as a mother
tongue) and two from Kerala (with Malayali). All but one spoke Tamil flu-
ently, but even she spoke well enough to get by. Unlike the major cities in
the north of India, where many of the sex workers are migrants from the
neighbouring countries of Nepal and Bangladesh (Ahmad 2005; Frederick
2005; Sleightholme and Sinha 2002), these waves of migrant women in sex
work had not reached Chennai (or my sample).

Again, religious background did not stop women from entering sex work, and all major religions were represented: mainly Hindu, but also Christians (four women) and Muslims (four women). Religion was signified by (for example) images of Hindu gods and Jesus on the walls of their homes, and in accessories, such as wearing a *pottu* (a red dot on the forehead, between the eyebrows) for Hindus, or not wearing one for Christians and Muslims. None of the Muslim women used the *burkha* (coverall coat) when they left the house. Going to a temple, mosque or church was often described as a way to give offerings to pray for a better future, and some women went to temple, mosque or church regularly, but none of the women represented themselves as overtly pious. Religion came across as a secular everyday practice. Four women self-defined themselves as multireligious, or having changed religion when they married, and they argued that all gods are the same.

Marital status, relationships and cohabitation

The marital careers of the women are the most sociologically interesting aspect of their socio-demographics. Their marital statuses, modes of cohabitation and amorous/erotic relationships challenge many dominant theories about south Indian gender relationships, and go a long way to help understand why and how the women had started to sell sex.

In Tamil Nadu, a woman can be married after she begins menstruating, and all the women I interviewed were of marriageable age. Their ages ranged from 14 to around 50, as shown in Table 3.1.

Three women were under 20 years of age (plus another two young women that I suspected or were rumoured to be under 20). Most (28) women were in their 30s, whereas the second-most prevalent age group was 20–29 years old (14 women). Two women were over 40 years old, and six were over 50. The low representation of minors in the sample should not be read as suggesting that under-age sex work does not exist. Such girls are very hard to reach, and are protected by the older women in their communities. Also, interestingly, the relatively large number of older sex workers problematises the idea of an age 'glass ceiling' for sex workers. However, my impression was that the oldest of these women were earning money predominantly by pimping rather than by selling sex.

Women's relationships were not so clear-cut that they could be easily divided between married and unmarried; their relationship histories were convoluted. Table 3.2 clarifies them and should be read against the existing assumptions of kinship, according to which women only live with (first) their parents, then (one) husband and, finally, their son, and the related norms about chastity and sexuality according to which they marry (in an arranged

Table 3.1 Women's ages

Age	Number of women
Below 20 years	3
20–29	14
30–39	28
40–49	2
Over 50	6
No answer	3
All women	56

Table 3.2 Domestic partners of all ever-married women

Domestic partner	Number of women
'Original' husband	18
Sister/other sex worker	8
Children/parents	9
Alone	3
Remarried/partner	8
No answer	1
All ever-married women	47
Unmarried	9

marriage) one man with whom they have sex (and are expected to have sex with no one else before or after that). The living and loving arrangements of the women in this research strikingly challenge these notions and clearly show that not all women in Chennai live according to these stereotypes.

Of the fifty-six sex workers, forty-seven were, or had been, married at some point in their life, whereas nine had never been married. The women's husbands were typically *kuli* (day labourer) workers, and were employed (for example) as autorikshaw drivers, construction workers, or fruit and vegetable sellers, or else they were unemployed.

Twelve marriages deviated from the norm of an arranged marriage. Ten women had eloped and made what is known locally as a 'love' marriage. This is a high number, given that arranged marriages are still customary in south India. The high incidence of women in sex work who have had a love marriage concurs with general understandings that options for women whose love marriage fails are limited, because of the stigma attached to love marriages, affecting the women concerned and their family honour (see Moody 2002). This stigma often leads to ostracism and lack of support from the woman's parents. In the other two cases, the women had married a man who had taken advantage of them sexually, whom they had then agreed to marry for the sake of their own and their family's honour. Ishika, for example, said that she had demanded this from her rapist, because she was afraid of being ostracised and to shield her family from shame.

The remaining thirty-five women's marriages were arranged as is the norm. Only two women mentioned having been married to a cross-cousin, a practice that was once customary in Tamil Nadu but now is less common. Their marriages had taken place when they were between the ages of 8 and 18, but the majority had wedded at around the age of 15. If the women had married young, they had fewer years of schooling, and if they had married later, it was more likely that they had attended a higher level of schooling (Table 3.3).

The normative expectation is of life-long marriage, and eighteen of the women were living with their first husband at the time of interview. Many of the original marriages – twenty-nine in fact – had then failed. When the women's marital statuses were not 'normative', who did they live with? In terms of cohabiting, as Table 3.2 shows, of the forty-seven women who were or had been married, twenty lived without a husband or partner at the time of my research. Of these twenty, eight lived with a sister or another female sex worker, nine lived with their own children or parents, and three lived completely alone.

In cases when marriages had come to an end, only Sheelamma's divorce from her husband was viewed positively by her in-laws, who gave her dowry back to ensure that her children received their inheritance. Later, once the rumours of her being in sex work came out, they resented Sheelamma bitterly. In most cases, if the women had lived together with their in-laws when the separation occurred, the women left their husbands and their in-laws did not ask them to come back (in fact, Sripriya's and Vasumathi's in-laws were responsible for ostracising them and throwing them out of the house, on the grounds that they both had a bad omen in their horoscopes). When the

Table 3.3 Years in school

Schooling experiences	Number of women
No schooling	4
1–2 years	0
3–4	1
5–6	8
7–8	7
9–10	7
11–12	1
No answer	28
All women	56

women left their husbands, it was clear that they did not want to continue living with them or their in-laws. But even if the women were left by their husbands, they complained that it was still difficult to go back to their natal home.

Women's chastity is related to marriage and, just as widows are seen as impure (Hancock 1999), women who have been married and fall out with their husbands can be seen to have transgressed the same boundaries of chastity and are not necessarily welcomed back to their families. Poor families, especially, are unable to take a daughter and her children back, as this would mean more mouths to feed. Sripriya recounts her experience: ' "Everything is over, you need to go now," they said. And they never gave food to my child and I was starving at my house and no one bothered to ask about me' (interview transcript: p. 3 lines 36–9, 25 April 2008).

A disproportionately large number of women in the sample had love marriages, and, particularly in those cases, when the marriages came to an end, the women were rejected by both their in-laws and their natal family. For example, Sangita married a non-Muslim man. He turned out to be very violent and also demanded that she should have sex with his friends. She ran away from him, but because of the shame of her love marriage, she was rejected by her sisters (both her parents had already died). This suggests that, after the marital break-up, most of these women were either forced or chose to live without their parents or in-laws – despite the fact that it is rare for women to live alone or without their families. In this way, natal families and in-laws contributed to the difficult situation in which these women had to face poverty: in more general terms, the decay of the family structure contributes to the pressures that funnel poor women towards sex work.

All of the women interviewed had partners, whether they lived alone or were in marital relationships. Eight women (Jayati, Sripriya, Sasika, Swasti, Sangita, Madhu, Lavali and Sindhu) had remarried or lived in a permanent relationship with a regular partner. 'Regular partner' here means someone who is regarded as permanent, not just as a regular client in sex work, although this line was sometimes blurred. Women in all of these statuses had sex with familiar customers for money. The regular partners were called *partners*, *lovers*, *boyfriends*, or, in some cases, the women referred to themselves as a *keep* (a kept woman), or as a second/third/fourth wife if they did not have a husband already. The comments suggested that a man could have several wives at one time, but these women never said that they had several 'husbands' simultaneously (even if they did).

These non-normative but fairly regular relationships were not confined to those whose marriages had broken up. Of the women who were still married to their initial husbands, eight of them (Uma, Mahadevi, Ishwari, Zaima, Ponni, Suddha, Diya and Jayati) had regular partners or boyfriends outside their marriages. According to the women concerned, in one-half of these cases their husbands did not have extramarital affairs. Seven women who lived alone (Revati, Sevati, Manjula, Bina, Vasumathi, Suwarna and Kanchi) had partners who did not cohabitate with them. The reasons given for this included: that the men had other wives; that marriage was seen as unsuitable (for example, if the woman was older); that the relationship was based on love (rather than being arranged) and there were no chances of it being arranged; or simply that they did not want to have a man around the house. Of the nine women who were not married, five were young (Maria, Sheila, Vanita, Pramila and Sonali), although not all were minors and they did not have regular partners. Two unmarried older women (Avantika and Revati) (one of whom was a *devadasi*) remained single, and two unmarried women (Manjula and Sevati) (one of whom was a *devadasi*) had regular partners but they were not cohabiting with them.

These findings highlight two things. First, women who had a 'deviant' role as a sex worker simultaneously made attempts to live according to normative expectations, in familial settings with a husband or a long-term partner. Swasti is an example of a woman whose initial marriage had broken up and who had remarried:

> I did not marry him for money or anything, I just married 'cos he approached me and asked me to get married to him. He's working in catering, cooks for weddings. He already has a wife … I'm just keeping him as a man in my life. Basically I need protection and want a man in my life. So he doesn't give me money but instead, sometimes, I have to give him some money. The only thing is that he takes care of the children and stays around and is a man in the house.
>
> (Interview transcript: p. 2, lines 2–4;
> p. 4, lines 32–5, 20 May 2005)

Second, despite the normative attempts, my findings suggest that these women had made choices about their relationships with the notion of 'desire' in mind – they were not asexual, and their relationships did not always aim at reproduction. As shown earlier, the rise of HIV has brought attention to sexual behaviour that is not confined to heteronormative monogamous relationships. This has meant addressing the issue of both men who have sex with men (MSM) and female sex workers. Although HIV prevention directed at female sex workers assumes heterosexual orientation, this was not the orientation of all the women that I interviewed.

Mercy, as we have seen, defined her sexual orientation as lesbian and two others (Zaima and Komala) had had bisexual experiences, whereas the remainder were either in heterosexual relationships or did not report same-sex relationships. The other women talked entirely about men as their partners, clients and objects of desire. Those who were asked about same-sex relationships either sneered at them or said they thought they were odd. Uma said that sometimes clients asked for group sex, but that she had never had sex with another woman. She said that there are a few lesbian women in the NGO office that she goes to: 'When I see them, I will tease them. It made me laugh to see people like that. That's why this country is getting bad' (interview transcript: p. 6, lines 30–41, 11 June 2005). There is no public discourse of female same-sex relationships in India, despite the controversial public attention brought to bear by the response to the art film *Fire* (1996). Rather than encouraging public debate concerning lesbian rights, *Fire* was represented as an 'inappropriate' film and shown in 'blue' film theatres as pornography. There were no lesbian organisations in Chennai to promote their rights, nor did the projects that dealt with MSM issues have this as part of their agenda. None of the three women concerned lived in a permanent relationship with a woman at the time of my research; Mercy had done so in the past but now lived alone, Zaima lived with her husband and children, and Komala lived with her son.

Three women – not originally from Chennai – were from *devadasi*[2] backgrounds. In two cases (Manjula and Avantika), they were not from *devadasi* families but instead had been 'married to the gods' as an offering when they were toddlers at the breakout of pestilences: in Manjula's case this was chickenpox, whereas cholera had affected Avantika's village. Neither had actually lived in a temple but, rather, the *devadasihood* had bound them only in that they were unable to marry. In the case of the third woman, Sripriya, her aunts on her father's side of the family had been *devadasis*. When she looked for a way to make money after her husband had abandoned her and when her father died, she was advised by her family that she could make money through sex because it was acceptable for them, as they were from a *devadasi* family. I asked Avantika if being a *devadasi* was positive or negative, to which she responded:

> I don't want marriage, all that, I'm happy. There is no problem. No one is asking questions. I have food, I'm happy. Whatever I can do ... If you have marriage, you will have so much trouble in your life. Being a *devadasi*, you are more happy. Without marriage you can have a happy life ... I was very happy to say I was a *devadasi*. I don't want that circle, husband, wife, that circle. I don't want to be money-minded. I can put on make-up; I can walk the main road. In a family, I cannot wear make-up, I cannot ... Cultural problem will come. I am happy like this. I don't want any relations, only friends. Only friends can help. All relations are money-minded.
>
> (Interview transcript: p. 6, lines 10–16, 20 February 2005)

Manjula and Sripriya, who both lived with partners, were more ambivalent about the status. Although stating that being a *devadasi* was not shameful, Manjula still suffered from not being able to marry properly, as she was the third wife of a man who was violent towards her, whereas Sripriya was now in a relationship that she was pleased with and had stopped doing sex work.

Devadasis provide ruptures in the discourse of womanhood that views women as essentially chaste and reproductive orientated. Evidence for this is provided in the accounts of two of the three *devadasis* that I had the chance to interview. Manjula had, by choice, not married, but now lived with a partner. Avantika had hoped to get married to a young man, but her being a *devadasi* had prevented that. They both pointed out that *devadasis* no longer dance at the temples, but that their right as a *devadasi* is that they can have sex with anybody they want without anybody being able to challenge them. Manjula in particular gave the impression that she felt very liberated by the fact that she did not have the responsibilities of housework or child care and she was not expected to follow the norms of female sexuality. These two women were able subvert the norms of chastity because of their *devadasi* background. This suggests that, in Tamil culture, there are groups to whom sex work is socially 'allowed'. Generally, *devadasi* is not seen as a positive role, and it is a role available only to those who have family ties to *devadasis* or who have had that role since childhood, which may help to explain why sex workers have not taken on this identity as a foundation of a social movement.

Sex work as a strategy against poverty

From a structural viewpoint, Indian society is often described as having distinctive roles for men and women, in which women stay at home and look after the household and children while men earn money and look after the family's income. The patriarchal ideal supposedly 'guarantees' that women will initially be looked after by their fathers, then by their husbands, and, finally, by their son(s). This distinctively sharp division between productive and reproductive labour can create problems, however, if the system fails (for example, due to financial reasons) – and, indeed, *purdah* is more strictly observed among families that can afford to keep their women at home (see Caplan 1985; Hancock 1999; Jeffery 1979; Trawick 1990). If women are forced to take on the role of maintaining the family – whether due to the collapse of the traditional arrangements or for other reasons – they usually have few resources, skills or training to help them to do so (and for a similar analysis of women in sex work in Calcutta, see Sleightholme and Sinha 2002). Therefore, these women shared class – rather than caste, ethnicity or religion – as their unifying socio-demographic characteristic.

In the interviews, sex work came across predominantly as a strategy to fight financial hardship. As Ishwari put it: 'I'm earning money for food' (interview transcript p. 2 line 28, 24 March 2005). Many of the women described how they did not have enough resources to survive and that they needed to make money by selling sex for survival and maintaining the family.

Leena:	My husband doesn't give anything; I have to put it all for the rent and pay the school fees … he'd go in the morning and return at 10 pm at night. With what he earns, it would just cover the price of coffee so that's why I put on a cotton sari and went to work as a housemaid. I didn't know about sex work. As a housemaid you get Rs. 300 … Then one day the man of the house called me and he locked the door. He said come to me and said: 'I'll give you Rs. 400' and asked me to make love on the house bed. That was the first I know of this work …
Salla:	After intercourse, how do you feel?
Leena:	It is difficult, we [I] never anticipated we'd [I] have to do this; we [I] came expecting our husbands to earn money for us. And it's really painful; if my husband is not about, I'll bathe it in hot water. We [I] suffer, oh, so much. And it really happens, but what to do? The family has to be saved … if I don't get Rs. 500 I myself will phone to make them [clients] come.

(Interview transcript: p. 3, lines 19–29;
p. 7, line 44; p. 8, line 2, 16 May 2005)

The women interviewed did not live in designated areas ('red light districts'), although groups of sex workers were able to live together if a non-judgemental landlord allowed this. The areas where the women lived within Chennai could be described as urban low-income ones; in some cases they lived in slightly improved squatter settlements, but generally they did not live in the worst areas of the town (which were usually located along the rivers of Chennai and near the beaches). The low-income areas in Chennai are scattered around the town, such as around Tondiarpet, Tiruvottiur and Erukkancheri in the north, Vadapazhani, Koyambedu, Kodambakkam in the west, K.K. Nagar and T. Nagar in the south-west, and Poorur, Poonamallee and Avadi at the edges of the town. The Tamil Nadu Slum Clearance Board has worked to upgrade the slums in Chennai. Houses are made of concrete, even if they sometimes have thatched roofs. Water is very sparse in Chennai, and the areas where the women lived had communal water pumps where the women collected water to be stored in their houses. All homes had electricity. The areas were cramped and lacked privacy, and families stayed in minute spaces where a room – sometimes less than two by five metres in size – was shared between as many as six people. Only a few had private toilet and washing spaces. Despite the cramped spaces and low income, many families had pets, such as ornamental fish, rabbits, dogs, pet rats, birds and boa snakes. Only Sindhamani owned a flat in a lower-middle-class area. The poorest huts were in reeking slums and made of coconut leaf, with a cardboard door and sleeping mats without any furniture or belongings.

Many women had come from poor families and, when they were young, there had been too many children, so daughters were married off at an early age. For example, Bina was married at the age of 13 and Madhu as early as 8. Kaveri explained that, in her family, there were four boys and four girls and that she had the main responsibility for housework because her mother was working outside the house. Food was always a problem, and she would often have to feed dinner to her siblings. Despite the hardships, she described a happy childhood. She was married around the age of 15 and commented that her life before marriage was harder than at present.

Not all the women were originally lower class, however, but something had happened in their lives that then led to poverty. In their biographies, for example, Sheelamma, Sindhu and Uma described how they had grown up in and/or married into privileged land-owning families. Sheelamma serves as an example: she was married to a man from a wealthy family in Kerala when she was 13, and her father gave her some sovereigns of gold to take with her. She and her husband had several servants: 'life was good'. However, after 7 years, her husband had an affair with one of the servant girls and got her pregnant. After serious fighting and domestic violence, Sheelamma obtained a divorce. When they divorced, her gold was divided between the children and, with that money, the children were educated in convents and now hold degrees in law, medicine, etc. Sheelamma, on the other hand, lives now in a dark, hot room that is 3 metres × 2 metres in size by herself, without any contact with her children. So, for her, as for many others, sex work served as a strategy to survive in difficult circumstances, and not only women who were 'originally' poor entered sex work.

Lower-caste and lower-class women have always worked in India, so this alone does not explain why some women but not others enter sex work; other factors must be involved as well. For these women, selling sex was a way to negotiate financial hardships, but was not always an act of desperation. The average price for sex among the women interviewed ranged between Rs. 100 and Rs. 250. Madhu, Chapala and Ishika charged the least – Rs. 20 (23p) – and also said that they occasionally sold blood to get money. A couple of young women said they would get about Rs. 1,000 (£11.50) per client. This suggests a huge variety in the contribution that sex work provided to the women's income. The possibility of earning relatively good money reasonably fast meant that sex work was not always a matter of survival. In a few cases, the women explained that sex work was also a practical way to gain more skills and to clear off debts. Ponni, for example, said that she wanted to help her husband start a business, and so took out Rs. 10,000 as a loan: 'But when I was unable to pay back the debt, the money lenders said "go and sleep with someone and get the money back" so I was able to clear that off' (interview transcript: p. 1 lines 13–14, 30 May 2005) Likewise, Neela tried to help her sister to get better job opportunities: 'I thought well of her and I put her in some dance class and paid Rs. 500 on her behalf' (interview transcript: p. 1 lines 39–40, 17 May 2005).

Most women explained sex work in terms of necessity. But were they hesitant to say they profited from sex work beyond obtaining 'necessities'? Perhaps because of the social stigma of sex work, very few women admitted that they used sex work to try to increase their life standards above a basic level. Potentially, sex work can be a lucrative business through which one could earn a lot of money – if one is fair-skinned, cunning and can attract rich clients – but this was rare. Only one woman managed this (and said it openly). She earned the highest monthly income: Rs. 10,000. This is approximately as much as a college-educated person can earn in an IT job in Chennai. She ran a souvenir shop to camouflage her earnings and to waive suspicions regarding her income. However, for most of the women, sex work was a backdoor option. Pooja explained that she knew that she could put on her most beautiful *sari* and go and stand at the bus stop if she needed money. Most women did not work full time, and sex work contributed only a part of their income. Nonetheless, poverty was reported as the foremost reason why women had needed to go out and look for jobs when the 'traditional' family structure had failed.

Failure of family structure: women as heads of households

Except for nine younger women, the rest of the women had been married before they started to work as sex workers. All of the married sex workers presented an account of how, in their particular cases, their family had failed them. Their husbands and fathers either could not, or chose not, to look after their financial needs and those of their families. These men had died, left, fallen sick, become unemployed, or had other wives, and thus their contribution to the household's income was insufficient or non-existent.

After my husband left me and I went to my mother's house, they told me that they can't take care of us all. I took my other child and was roaming around – what can you do with a baby in your arm? I even begged and I was crying and praying …

(Neela – interview transcript: p. 1, lines 22–4, 17 May 2005)

The married women who cohabited with their husbands (such as Suddha, Kuntala, Uma, Sharita, and Ishwari) said that they had started sex work because their husbands did not have a job and therefore their families did not have money for food and bills. Their husbands worked in *kuli* (day labour) jobs whenever there was work available, but, commonly, the men had work less than once a week and this was not enough to cover the family's expenses. Men were often described as 'no good' and irresponsible and this was interpreted as a lack of love or caring on their part. Ponni and Leena said that their husbands did not give them money to run the household, although they earned some money themselves. Similarly, the husbands of Kuntala, Sangita, Jayati and Maya did earn money, but used their earnings to buy alcohol or drugs, and Jayati and Maya eventually grew tired of it and left them. Because of this, the women said, they were forced to look after themselves and their families by whatever means that they had.

While blaming their husbands for the collapse of the family's living situation underpins this narrative, it was not always the men who initiated the break-up. Of those women who were separated from their husbands, in at least seven cases the women had left their husbands. Some had left because of his drug and alcohol use (Maya, Sangita and Jayati); some (Sangita, Swasti, Jayati, Sheelamma and Bina) also said that they had left because of domestic violence: Swasti effectively threw out her husband after she grew tired of domestic violence. Some (Sharita, Vasumathi and Sheelamma) left because their husbands had brought a second wife to the house. 'I left him. He gave me trouble, beating me, torturing me, took drugs so I left him … It was really difficult with him beating me and that, so I came away by myself (Jayati – interview transcript: p. 1, lines 24–6, 3 April 2005). 'After 5 years of domestic violence I told him: "Why don't you go to your first wife? I can't tolerate this anymore" ' (Swasti – interview transcript: p. 1, lines 27–8, 20 May 2005).

These experiences show that women have more agency in household matters than characterisations of victimhood and arguments about women's powerlessness in household relationships might suggest. However, effectively, although not necessarily directly, the women were involved in creating the situation that led them to sex work. Ironically, when women sought to get out of violent and abusive relationships, they fell into other circumstances that were also violent and abusive. Their decisions were in most cases driven by concern of their children, and motherhood and its requirements was a dominant explanation of why they got into selling sex.

Motherhood

Marriage in Tamil culture is associated with children, and all of the married women had them. Besides poverty, and the collapse of the patriarchal family system, another pervasive explanation for women being involved in sex work was to take care of their children. The women had one to five children, most often two or three, after which they had undergone sterilisation, the commonest form of birth control in Tamil Nadu. The nine unmarried women did not have children, but reported abortions. Four women reported that they had had babies that had died or were stillborn, but this number could be higher because I asked only about living children and the women tended to disclose infant deaths or stillbirths only if it had been particularly traumatic for them. The general reproductive period in the women's lives was between 13 and 24. Those under the age of 18 who had children had them either living with them or, in three cases, had put them to live in a hostel. Women in the older age groups (above 40) had children who were married, many of whom, according to the women, did not keep in touch with them. All the women talked about their children and motherhood came across as a very strong positive identity – but sustaining the children was also a strong reason why the women did sex work.

Income from other sources was simply not enough to cover the costs of the children's school fees, books, clothes and so on. Some of the women had put their children into an 'English' school to ensure that they would learn English properly and thus get a better education and better future opportunities. In this way, educating their children was an investment – almost the only one available to them. Some women gave their children away to be looked after by a relative, or sent them to a boarding school to be educated. The importance of motherhood explains why these women take chances at the expense of their own health and safety.

> He was a drug addict and I left him. At that point of time I had to take care of all the needs and necessities of my children … I want my way of life to end with me and I don't want my children to get into it. They should never know about my secret [about sex work] and I want to end my life like that. My children's future will be spoiled because they are grown now, I should be a good mother. If I am not a good mother then they might ask me 'Are you a mother, you do a whore's job?' In Tamil this is how they will say. They won't ask me if they brought me by this work.
>
> (Maya – interview transcript: p. 2,
> lines 12, 22–3, 11 May 2005)

After the marriage and after my husband left me I entered into this for the sake of my children. I should support my children … I want my children to progress in life.

(Sripriya – interview transcript: p. 2, lines 10–11;
p. 8, line 50, 25 April 2005)

Salla: Do you love him [a regular customer/lover]?
Kaveri: His caste is different. He is a Muslim. I'm a different caste. We see each other, speak and go for the odd trips, but that's it. I'm doing it for money. I like him but he's not that handsome. He has a different personality; I just do it for my kids.

(Interview transcript: p. 5, lines 25–7, 17 June 2005)

Family situations were such that the women needed to contribute to the household earnings in order to provide for their children: a rationale that could be another acceptable discourse for women to explain their actions. The marriage system around the women had eroded for one reason or another, and they were left alone to look after themselves and their children. Although these women were unable to meet societal expectation as wives, acting according to their female gender role and looking after their children was still acting according to the norms of the society. In explaining that they entered sex work because of their children, they emphasised the altruistic role of a mother. The majority of the women did live with their children, though five of them had sent their children to be looked after by in-laws or in hostels. If there had been a greater number of women without their children, this would have ruptured the discourse of motherhood, but this still would not necessarily suggest that those women who had given their children away were 'un-motherly', as the wider society often regarded them. That is, giving children away was often described in relation to the fact that there was not enough money in the house and that the children were considered to receive better education in the hostels or with relatives.

When women made references in the interviews to motherhood, this could be seen as an attempt to construct a more positive identity. Identity as a mother offered them a chance to manage the negative role they had as a sex worker. And by doing so, the women were also tapping into the Tamil national discourse of women as mothers and self-sacrificing, and indicating that they were still good mothers and women: even if they were acting against the norm of chastity, after all, they were doing it for their children. And at the same time, this could also be an attempt to externalise the 'fault' or the 'misbehaviour' and assign responsibility to the men and to external structures, thereby removing it from themselves.

Accounts that emphasise motherhood illustrate how normative, in Tamil Nadu, is the woman's role as a wife and a mother. Not all of the women, however, wanted the role of a woman who stays in the house, looking after the children. In particular, Kuntala and Maya felt that they were trapped in their homes and they looked for company outside. This did not turn out as they expected, because they ended up doing sex work, but it still shows ruptures in the discourse of women's feelings and attitudes towards their given role as women. These examples also challenge the passive representation of women to sexuality: at times they initiated the very relationships that led them to having sex with men for money.

> I didn't have anybody to talk to about my husband and problems. Both my sister were like that, asocial or mental. I was social but there was no company, I was unable to be myself or free. When I tried to look for company from outside, other people pulled me into this. I needed support and companionship but they turned out bad.
>
> (Kuntala – interview transcript: p. 3, lines 47–51, 11 May 2005)

> One of my friends saw that I was fed up with life and I was very young, I would have been 22 or 23 years. My friend said that I have to enjoy life and she made me meet a guy, that is, as a love affair, and then I entered into this path step by step.
>
> (Maya – interview transcript: p. 2, lines 17–20, 11 May 2005)

Employment opportunities for women

The women explained that, prior to starting, and alongside, doing sex work, they also worked at some of the other jobs that are generally available to uneducated labourers – for example, as construction workers, guards, export factory workers or maids.[3] They were able to get only these jobs because their education level was not high and they did not have the skills that would have enabled them to get better paying ones. Their education level varied from no schooling to the twelfth standard (see Table 3.3). One sex worker (not part of the sample, because I was unable to interview her properly) was the lead peer educator in an HIV prevention NGO just outside Chennai: she had a college education. Four women had not attended school at all. The second major cut-off point was after the fifth standard (class), when primary school is completed. Eight of the women had studied up to fifth to sixth standard. Seven had studied to seventh to eighth standard, seven women up to ninth to tenth standard and one woman reported having completed twelfth standard. Twenty-eight women did not disclose their education level.

Education among these women was higher than reported by the APAC, which funds NGOs with aid given by USAID and provides statistics about sex workers in Tamil Nadu. According to APAC (2005b), one-third of the female sex workers in six cities in Tamil Nadu were illiterate, and forty-seven per cent had completed primary education (up to class five). Even if most of the women interviewed for this research who disclosed their level of education had schooling, there were still some who did not know how to read or write. They could write their own name and all of them knew basic maths – for instance, to calculate how much they had been cheated if the client did not pay as originally agreed. Three women (Pugazh, Maya and Zaima) understood a little English. The interviews do not provide evidence that would suggest a connection between the level of education and the ability to negotiate sex work to one's benefit or avoid the violence related to sex work. Lack of education in, and of, itself does not lead to sex work. Instead, education combined with other factors such as the break-up of marriage, poverty and a limited number of options for employment made sex work a viable option to earn money.

Opportunities for unskilled, often illiterate, women are limited, and finding a job that would cover the expenses of a family with several children was difficult. The women stated that they entered sex work for their and their families' survival, because their initial jobs were not enough to run the family. When they had been working in other jobs, all of the women reported that men had harassed them sexually (similar findings about women's experiences of sexual harassment in the work place have been reported from Chennai by Swaminathan 2004). From this, they said, it was a small step to sex work. They had to decide between a low-paying job in which they received sexual abuse, and higher paying sex work, which meant more money with less effort.

> I saw that wherever I went it was like that, housemaid work, company work – there you had to 'adjust' and work otherwise you'd not get the job, then you'll get Rs. 1,000 salary – how many would I have to adjust to? Ten people – can I do that? They do pay although some cheat on you, say they love you – you can't trust anyone these days. So with sex work you get a phone call, go to their house and get Rs. 500 in hand and you arrange with two or three people. If I don't have work, I'll stay at home.
>
> (Vanita – interview transcript:
> p. 3, lines 31–6, 16 May 2005)

For some women, there had been ignorance or a misunderstanding of the nature of what was being suggested to them. Pooja's husband fell sick, she tried to borrow money from her friend and then:

> The friend asked why Pooja wanted to get into debt; she knew a way to make money for free: 'Come tomorrow wearing your best dress.' The lady took her to a lodge at Kovalam beach to see a client. Pooja hesitated but the agent persuaded her: 'You have already come here, why should you not do it? If you go home now, your husband will ask you where you have been the whole day and you come in empty handed. Anyway you have been inside the lodge and your reputation is spoilt when people see you coming out.'
>
> (Field notes: 28 October 2004)

As in the case of Pooja, madams often had a role in bringing women into sex work. Muyal said: 'There was no livelihood. I went to the cinema and there were female agents who said you can get money and don't have to suffer any more' (interview transcript: p. 9, lines 26–35, 24 May 2005). Her comment suggests that madams network women and clients. However, this relationship did not always require coercion. Ponni herself had approached one of the madams in her neighbourhood:

> Six months ago there was a problem in the home and there was no money so I actually asked one of the ladies here who is also a sex worker about some job – 'Is there any work in here?'
>
> (Interview transcript: p. 4, lines 17–19, 30 May 2005)

Based on accounts such as this, it would be one-dimensional to suggest that all women were tricked or coerced into sex work, or that they lacked agency. Neela provides an example of making the decision to enter sex work:

> My husband abandoned me so I had to look for an outside job. I worked in government jobs [as a cleaner] and at construction sites. Everywhere I went there were men who asked for sex from me. At some point I thought, why would I not make money that way rather than burden myself at these tiring jobs?
>
> (Field notes: 18 May 2005)

Another example of an 'easy career choice' decision came from Sripriya. Her husband deserted her because of a bad omen in her horoscope – that the husband would be killed if a son was to be born in a certain month. She moved back to her parents' house but eventually her father fell ill and she needed to make more money for the family:

> When my father fell sick, at that time one lady approached me. I went there, I went for Rs. 5,000 and then I had been there for 1 month. That is a place where the brothel is. I was there for 1 month with the lady and I earned a lot of money … [However,] there were many raids and *rowdies* [causing] problems so after some time I left the brothel house. I came home and without depending on anybody I started to do the profession on my own.
>
> (Interview transcript: p. 5, lines 9–14, 44–47, 25 April 2005)

Apart from household jobs, factory work and construction site work, some of the women interviewed had worked in the film industry. From the women's accounts of their employment, trading sex seems to be strongly embedded within the film industry. The 'road to riches' story of a girl finding stardom through the film industry seems globally ubiquitous, and the film industry, *cini field*, is very important in the Chennai economy. Many films are made locally and require vast numbers of supporting actors and actresses. There was an expectation that women in supporting roles should have sex with the directors, managers, etc. in order to be recognised and to get a proper role. Madhu once told me: 'If the woman is in the *cini field*, it means she is a prostitute, she *has to* do that. It is a rule' (interview transcript: p. 6 lines, 14–15, 31 May 2005).

Responding to the sexual requests of men in the film industry was not restricted to those women who wanted their faces on the screen; those who wanted to get jobs in preparing the stars (for example, make-up artists) were also told that they had to use their bodies to climb the occupational ladder. Mercy used this opportunity to make contacts and promote her beauty parlour. A similar account is given by Zaima:

> It was fun [working as a make-up artist in the film industry] but we also needed to do this [sex] work and adjust with them. I got into this work by that and I did not enter into this willingly.
>
> (Interview transcript: p. 5, lines 38–9, 12 May 2005)

These accounts problematise the definition of sex work: the exchange of sex to get a role or position in a new film can also be defined as a kind of sex work. Furthermore, the same madams who recruited sex workers also recruited supporting actresses for the film industry. This suggests that the film industry and the sex trade are intimately inter-linked, which raises opportunities for future research.

Although many women were not pleased or happy about being in sex work, to see sex workers as victims is oversimplified. The accounts given above suggest that once a woman is in the sex industry, the quick and easy way it provides for making money becomes an incentive to stay in sex work – and this is not necessarily a 'disempowering' solution. The reasons and conditions that the women described as leading them to selling sex were oftentimes very harsh and left the women lacking in options. Still there was some amount of deliberation and agency involved. Actual coercion or trafficking was rare in my sample, although not unheard of.

Forced into selling sex

Trafficking – defined as someone being kidnapped and forced to work as a sex slave – was not observed or reported during my fieldwork. Despite the massive literature on trafficking and the moral panic about women being sold as sex slaves, as well as the reputation of India receiving sex slaves from her neighbouring countries (particularly Nepal and Bangladesh), active coercion was remarkably rarely mentioned by the women I interviewed as part of the route that had taken them into sex work. This may, of course, be because those women who have been trafficked are better protected, or because Chennai does not have a red light district (an easy target for trafficking) or mass brothels.

Four of the women (Swasti, Komala, Revati and Vasumathi), however, had been actively forced into sex work. Swasti was forced into sex work when she was looking for a job. She was approached by two women who told her about a household job for 2 weeks and offered her Rs. 1,500. She did not know it would entail sex work. In the job, she refused to have sex but ended up being beaten and tortured for her refusal. She told me that she had to host at least ten men a day and was sometimes locked in during the night. When she left after 2 weeks – it was unclear why she was able to leave at this point and not earlier – she discovered that she was pregnant and had an abortion because she felt she could not afford to have another child, but also because she believed that if her family found out about what happened they would kill her. Komala was also forced into sex work when she was looking for a job as a maid in Indonesia. Both of these women ended up in sex work after receiving false promises about work when they needed it. After the initial event, both of the women continued to work as sex workers independently.

Revati told me her life story, which was particularly gruesome. She was an orphan and at a young age was adopted by a woman who was a pimp.

After she reached puberty, her virginity was sold a to a man who was much older than her. After this, she stated that she was sold to various brothels around the country and was often drugged when she had her clients. All protestation or defiance resulted in a beating, and she commented that girls sometimes 'disappeared'. She also described raids that the police conducted to abolish mass brothels, and how they had to hide in a well behind the brothel so that the police could not find them. Eventually, she escaped with the help of a client, and at the time of the interview she lived alone with her daughter outside Chennai and supported herself by doing sex work independently. Vasumathi's husband, who turned out to be a pimp, forced her into sex work by first making her sleep with his friends and then blackmailing her to provide them with a more luxurious lifestyle. Vasumathi was the only woman with whom the husband was directly involved in the coercion or pimping. In her case, the socio-cultural pressures of servitude towards husbands made her accept her husband's coercion. Both Revati and Vasumathi also continued in sex work.

In several cases, exposure to other sex workers and accumulated poverty led women from the same family to go into sex work. In one family, the mother-in-law and her two daughters-in-law were sex workers and, in four cases, two sisters worked together. Three pairs of mothers and children were in sex work: Zaima's mother had been a sex worker; Sasika and Vanita worked together; Joshita (one of the above daughter-in-laws) did sex work and there was a rumour that her minor-aged daughter did too. I suspected a fourth pair: Bina was a peer educator who was always very ambivalent about her sex-work status, and I wondered if her daughter might also do sex work – she was a dancer. Rather than necessarily leading to the conclusion that this is a common practice, the finding that women from the same families had entered sex work could be due to the networks that I had access to, or it could suggest that women of the same families enter sex work due to desensitisation of the norms restricting this behaviour. Whatever the case may be, it neither supports the view that sex workers force their children to also become sex workers, as suggested by the documentary *Born into Brothels*, nor does it deny it, as suggested by Pardasani (2005) (both concerning Calcutta).

A young, unmarried woman's reputation strongly affects her marital opportunities, and some of the unmarried women – although not all of them – were minors. In Western sex-work theorising, being a minor is seen as a factor that makes the act of sex work inherently coercive. This needs to be considered with reference to marriage in the Tamil cultural context, however, where the acceptable marriageable age is much below 18. Minor girls were generally carefully protected by their madams (mothers, sisters or other older women from the community), so that I did not have a chance to interview many of them. Of the unmarried women, I was able to properly interview two (Vanita, 17 years old, and Sevati, 29 years old) and one, briefly (Pramila, 20 years old). I also attended home visits with NGO staff in which the status of another three girls became apparent (Sonali – about 20 years old, Maria – 18 years old, and Sheila –14 years old). I had doubts about two more young women who are not in my sample because of their undisclosed status, but they were the daughters of sex workers/peer educators that I knew well (Bina's daughter – 18 years old, and Joshita's daughter – about 12 years old); there were rumours that they had entered sex work, although this was never openly disclosed.

Vanita, who is 17 years old and has worked as a sex worker for 2 years, told me:

> Some come into sex work as 14-year-old girls as *akka* [Salla, lit. 'big sister'] knows, small girls. Can you classify 14 as small? Well, it's not eight, is it? [laughs]. But it's not like that, I mean that even for a 17- or 18-year-old who can start a family, she shouldn't go nor be in that field but she is. If she hasn't started a family, she is fresh.
>
> (Interview transcript: p. 9, lines 14–17, 16 May 2005)

Vanita is suggesting here that at the age of 17 to 18 women are considered old enough to get married (and thus to have sex), and that 14-year-olds are not children anymore, as they have usually reached puberty by then. However, she hesitates and finds it difficult to draw the line between being too young and being old enough to start sex work. By that definition, Vanita herself started doing sex work at a dubious age (15). I asked her how she thought sex work might affect her future marriage prospects and she explained that she was aware of how to act properly on her wedding night to protect her secret, saying, 'If I get married they'll know, because they'll think it [vagina] is loose. My friends, they tell me how to act, to say it hurts …' (interview transcript: p. 10 lines, 16–17, 16 May 2005).

Technically, except for Sheila and Joshita's daughter, the unmarried women were of a marriageable age and were not culturally considered to be 'too young'. The two older unmarried women, Sevati and Pramila, lived alone and did not have an aura of secrecy around them, as the rest of the girls who lived with their families certainly did. For example, Vanita's mother routinely lied about Vanita's age to me and to the NGO staff (whereas, to clients, she was presented as younger). Judging by the protection and secrecy around them, the people involved knew that others might think that having young girls in sex work is unacceptable, and several of the sex workers made negative comments about Vanita's mother:

Do you know Vanita and Sasika? The little girl and the mother? She does a lot. She goes without condoms. She actually has white discharge. A mother should not involve her daughter in to this business. She has only one daughter and even she will tell a customer for Vanita. They go for shooting, they go here and there, and, what, still they don't have money?! You should not involve your daughter into this, it is very unfair. Until you have married your daughter you should look after her very well. You should not leave your daughter and eat with that money.

(Swasti – interview transcript:
p. 5, lines 17–24, 20 May 2005)

Swasti suggests here that, despite the fact that some minor girls did sex work with their mothers, this was seen to be out of order. Many women specifically said that they would not allow their daughters to do sex work.

Notes on agency

The findings reported in this chapter complement existing knowledge regarding sex workers in Chennai and India. Currently, the dominant representation of sex workers comes from the HIV discourse: this suggests a health-orientated view of sex workers and presents them as victims of poverty and patriarchy, which drives them into sex work, making them vulnerable to HIV, and further violence and oppression. Viewed this way, these women are seen simply as victims in need of empowerment. However, the findings of my research, which begin to unfold in this chapter, show that the HIV-driven representation is a simplification the complex realities of the lives and careers of sex workers and does not properly account for the diversity of the group of the women involved.

Sex-working women used agency, albeit in rather limited circumstances. As others (see, for example, Blanchard *et al.* 2005; O'Neil *et al.* 2004; Sleightholme and Sinha 2002) suggest, poverty is often the main reason behind sex work. These women asserted the same, and they were all poor at the time of my research. Poverty is seen as related to a lack of education of women and thus a lack of options. The four detailed life stories are painful to read, because they highlight the oppressiveness of the lives of the sex workers; violence was experienced by many of them both when doing sex work and at home, and thus violence was not limited to women's roles as sex workers. For example, Zaima had to learn to deal with having been raped, along with experiences of marginalisation, abandonment and ostracism from her family. Yet, my respondents were generally more educated than those in the research conducted by APAC (2005b), which challenges the assumptions that only the poorest, uneducated women enter sex work.

Research in Calcutta (Sleightholme and Sinha 2002) suggests that a majority (albeit an unspecified percentage) of the women there were coerced, tricked or sold into sex work, often by a family member. Many women in Chennai had been in a situation in which their options were limited and they resorted to selling sex due to financial burdens, collapse of the family support system or coercion. Like Mercy and Kuntala, many had a chance to consider the idea among other options.

The framework of these interviews was undoubtedly influenced by my theoretical approach, the questions that I asked and how I asked them. This framework was influenced by the literature on sex workers' movements in the global North, which insist on sex workers' human rights and operate on the presumption that sex work is work, rather than a form of oppression. Simultaneously, it was informed by post-structuralist feminism (for example, Mahmood 2005), emphasising that agency is action, not just resistance, and by my wish to find ways to allow the sex workers to talk about their sexuality, a taboo topic. I was interested in studying these complexities further.

On the one hand, the interviews clearly show that the women faced violence and structural struggles. On the other, it was not difficult to identify signs of agency and resistance. All of the women displayed agency in some part of their lives – much more than any of the literature around gender in South Asia suggests. Mercy decided to start her own beauty parlour. Zaima had affairs with women. Uma had a boyfriend before marriage, as well as after marriage. Kuntala had looked for an extramarital affair because she was lonely and longed for company. These are striking examples of autonomy and individuality that contradict the stereotypes of women in India as submissive and passive. Agency and resistance were also present in stories in which women challenged their roles as obedient and chaste wives and mothers, and when they were sexually active to various degrees. The women were exposed to poverty as a result of failures of the family system, and they needed to work to support their children; they experienced sexual harassment at work and coercion, but, at the same time, they also made active decisions to continuing sex work independently. Also, for example, as noted in her life story, Zaima provided four different reasons for how she got into sex work: (1) through her mother pimping her before her maturity; (2) because they were poor; (3) by her neighbour pimping her when she was in a financially dire situation; and (4) because she needed contacts in the film industry when her marriage failed. In another example, Sripriya said in the beginning of her interview, 'I do this for my children' (interview transcript: p. 2, lines 10–11, 25 April 2005), but later on told me how she started to do sex work because her family was from a *devadasi* origin. These women, while they were bound by the structures of a non-individualist society in which women typically depend on men, had been forced to negotiate their lives on their own. The examples are evidence of how oppressive structures are managed in the lives of individuals through ways that, at times, are self-destructive and harmful, and at other times are positive and even subversive.

4 What happened to 3.2 million people?

HIV prevention – the main public arena in which sex work is addressed in Chennai – involves a variety of internationally funded government and NGO projects. Despite the considerable size of the expenditures involved, and many official reports, academic literature gives little insight into how these projects are conceptualised and implemented. This chapter provides a 'bottom-up' view of the relationships between global actors (such as the World Bank, UNAIDS and USAID), the Indian government, grass roots NGOs, and the targets of the interventions in the field – the sex workers themselves. These relationships have become an arena of development politics in which struggles for funds, resources, and identities are conducted.

In order to understand the need to adopt this approach, one needs to understand a pivotal moment in the representation of the situation of HIV in India. In May 2006, 20 years after the first case of HIV was discovered in India, UNAIDS (2006) announced that India had – at 5.7 million people – the highest number of people with HIV infections in the world. In 2007, using data collected using new methodologies, the United Nations estimate of HIV-positive people dropped to 2.5 million (UNAIDS 2007). Ethnographic and qualitative interview data from my fieldwork shed light on how and why both sets of numbers were produced. They suggest that HIV prevention programmes have become overzealously based on targets and numbers, leading to the use of incentives to attract 'new cases'. According to these data, NGOs' funding was tied to monitoring procedures that encouraged NGOs to inflate the numbers of female sex workers they contacted. Also, the women themselves used these NGOs as a form of livelihood, which may help to explain the inconsistencies between the two figures.

For the sex workers, the NGOs offered opportunities for mobilisation and the subversion of the stigmatised role as a sex work. But before such desired outcomes can be achieved, the NGOs and their daily working procedures also produce and reproduce existing inequalities. In Chennai, for instance, HIV prevention NGOs have failed to address sex workers' human rights or the structural asymmetries of power. The existing power hierarchies in the field, and the detachment of the global HIV prevention principles from the everyday experiences of the sex workers, undermine attempts to curb the spread of HIV. The attempts to empower sex workers have been laudable but ineffective because they have failed to address gender power imbalances and the poverty that drives women to sex work. These are the main factors that prevent sex workers from being able to negotiate condoms, let alone contribute to generating universal HIV awareness. This chapter begins by describing the HIV prevention programmes in India more broadly then narrows down to HIV prevention NGOs in Chennai more specifically, and, finally, presents five points that illustrate the above arguments in detail.

HIV prevention in India

Following structural adjustments in India, the Indian government has a decentralised, albeit dysfunctional, social welfare and health-care system. Charitable societies and non-governmental organisations play a major role in filling its gaps, in India in general and also (despite its reputation of having better health services than other parts of the country) in Tamil Nadu (see, for example, Caplan 1985). NGOs are seen to be well connected and capable of networking many people quickly. Since the finding of the first case of HIV in 1986 in Chennai, HIV prevention has become a major target of international aid and development work implemented by the NGOs.

The wider HIV prevention programme is coordinated by the National AIDS Control Organization (NACO) (National AIDS Control Organisation), a government body. NACO complies with the global guidelines that are set out and advocated by UNAIDS, as well as other organisations, such as the World Bank and USAID (retrieved on 21 October 2008 via: www.nacoonline.org/Partnerships/Donor_Partners/). NACO gets most of its funding for HIV prevention from the World Bank, but also from other organisations such as the Department for International Development (DFID) and USAID, and then distributes funds to state-level organisations. In 2004–05, NACO received Rs. 442.19 crore (= Rs. 4.42 billion = £55.22 million), most of which came from the World Bank.

Within Tamil Nadu, the HIV/AIDS 'problem' has become so focused on Chennai that the city has its own HIV prevention body – Chennai AIDS Prevention and Control Society (CAPACS). In 2004–05, Ahmedabad and Mumbai were the only other Indian cities to have their own societies.

Additionally, HIV prevention activities in Chennai, Tamil Nadu and Pondicherry (a separate state from Tamil Nadu but often attached to Tamil Nadu HIV prevention projects) are funded by APAC and the Tamil Nadu AIDS Initiative (TAI). APAC funds over sixty projects and is supported directly from USAID; TAI (supporting over twenty-five projects across Tamil Nadu) receives funds from the Bill and Melinda Gates Foundation, which they then distribute to the NGOs that work in the field. CAPACS funds fifteen projects in Chennai.[4] Other independent funding bodies were the Elton John Foundation, Johns Hopkins University, ActionAid and several smaller donors in Europe. During my fieldwork, I discovered that many NGOs received money from all of these sources. Grants were given for condom promotion, for the development of voluntary testing centres, to promote behaviour change and to train health experts. But there was no money to fund the immediate, often social–economic needs of high-risk groups that might make a sex worker have to accept a client without a condom when more money is offered. HIV was treated as a health, not a social problem.

This chapter discusses records of participant observation and interviews in six NGOs across Chennai. The NGOs worked mostly with female sex workers, but also with MSM. These NGOs had different organisational histories in social welfare and health care; for example, one had started as an NGO that helped blind people. Their commitment to HIV work seemed also to be conditional: after the 2004 tsunami, almost all the NGOs shifted to tsunami relief. While Tamil Nadu certainly suffered from the tsunami, the shift to tsunami relief had more to do with the availability of international funding than to the scale of the social problems it caused. This reflects the precariousness of funding for NGOs, and later in the chapter I will return to this issue when discussing the use of incentives and quotas in HIV prevention. In order to secure their funding, NGOs have to follow the global trends in aid and thus operate within the financial environment available to them. In order to attract these funds, they need to maintain a certain rhetoric to appeal to the funding bodies (for a similar argument elsewhere in the development sector, see Mosse 2005). I quote my field notes for a cynical interpretation of the situation:

> CAPACS consultant Ms Mathu said that NGOs merely keep up their own reputation and position rather than the cause of the sex workers. She argued that NGOs are not necessarily corrupted and greedy but do so to gain status and steady income: 'When one has skills to apply for money, it comes in; the funding bodies do not measure how much one loves the job or how sympathetic one is to the target group.'
>
> (Field notes: 4 April 2005)

The NGOs generally followed the national and global guidelines and were funded from the same sources; thus they were very similar in everyday practice. The main mode of HIV prevention used by NGOs in Chennai was the recruitment of 'peer educators', vocal and powerful individuals chosen from among the 'target group' to communicate with other sex workers (the role of peer educators will be elaborated later). NGOs' activities also included organising meetings for the sex workers, smaller ones weekly or monthly, larger ones annually; occasional special events targeted at the general public and stakeholders related to sex work, such as doctors, lawyers or other civil society representatives. One example was the showing of a documentary about HIV patients in Tamil Nadu. Similarly, on World AIDS Day, most NGOs organised demonstrations. NGOs varied considerably in their ability to arrange these events, some being haphazardbut others very organised.

NGOs were mostly located in middle-class areas, and spread their activities across the city rather than focusing on a particular location. Some had immaculate, air-conditioned offices that were well equipped with the most recent computer technology in upper-class neighbourhoods, whereas others were in rather shabby parts of town, poorly maintained, dirty and shady. In the absences of a red light district in Chennai, these NGOs were not necessarily in the areas where the sex workers lived, nor exactly where sex took place: these sites are also spread across the city. Generally, the NGO premises had several rooms with desks and plastic chairs. No matter how small the NGO, project coordinators had their own rooms. Apart from one NGO that was associated with a hospital, the NGOs had no medical facilities.

What generally characterised the outlook of the NGOs were condom promotion adverts on the walls, hand-made maps and charts, and campaigning posters. The hand-made maps were 'deviance maps' of Chennai, references to where sex work took place. They identified spots of sex work: pick-up points and where sex was bought and sold. Charts outlined how many condoms had been distributed, how many new contacts had been made with sex workers and how many people had been advised for testing. These were visible signs for guests of the work that the NGOs did, and were often shown as evidence of the NGOs' activities. Later in the fieldwork I observed that charts tended to reflect the promises that NGOs had made in their submissions to their funding bodies. The condom adverts and campaigning posters were cartoons with text in Tamil and English that encouraged people to practise safe sex. These adverts and posters summarised symptoms and ways of spreading HIV and STDs. In a sex workers' project, the posters had pictures of women with men; in an MSM project, the pictures were of effeminate men with masculine partners. Some posters promoted abstinence and being faithful before using condoms; these were distributed by APAC, and were funded by USAID, and therefore reflected the US government's ABC policy (Abstinence, Be faithful, use Condoms).

Some sex workers described these pictures as impure and inappropriate, and they did not want to visit the NGOs and have to look at them. Similar information was available in IE (Information and Education) leaflets available in most offices. Condoms were available in most offices on request rather than being openly on display. During the entire year I only witnessed one woman once asking for condoms. This might be coincidental, or it could mean that because women could not discreetly pick them up but had to ask for them the embarrassment might have stopped them from doing so.

There are no distinct places for sex workers to interact in Chennai, and anonymity from their neighbours and communities is very important to the women. NGOs provided such a space: sex workers could spend time, meet other women and relax. This was usually in a rather empty space without much furniture; people sat on the floors on mats and cushions. A few offices had a TV in this room. Although most offices offered tea to everybody in the afternoon, some also offered *'meals'* (rice and curries). Some offered food in weekly meetings, whereas some only provided lunch if there was a larger meeting, the kind that took place once every couple of months. For many of the women, food was an important part of the incentive to come to the NGO offices.

Despite being nominally organisations *for* sex workers, then, the NGOs were not run *by* them. Sex workers only visited the NGOs when they could receive some benefits – social, personal or economic. How, then, was HIV prevention performed in practice in these organisations? HIV prevention practices were a collaborative performance, by NGOs and by sex workers who became peer educators. Peer educators played key roles, embodying and reproducing the rhetoric of HIV prevention, and carefully deploying incentives to attract other sex workers. Such approaches meant that HIV prevention was double edged: it provided women with opportunities for social mobilisation, gaining funds and the subversion of the stigma on sex work, but taking part in these activities also reinforced their marginality.

Peer education and HIV prevention

Particular models and methods in HIV prevention have travelled globally and are used internationally (Karnik 2001; Treichler 1999). An example of this is the use of peer educators (for Thailand and the Philippines, see Murray and Robinson 1996; for South Africa, see MacPhail and Campbell 2001; for Tanzania, see Laukamm-Josten *et al.* 2000; for India, see Asthana and Oostvogels 1996; Dandona *et al.* 2005). All of the organisations that I visited used peer educators to find and recruit new sex workers for the NGOs' networks, directing sex workers to voluntary counselling and testing at the government hospitals, counselling in general, distributing condoms, doing social marketing of condoms to local shops, and attending awareness-raising events targeted at stakeholders. Peer educators were well connected among the sex workers because they were or had been in the past 'madams' – brokers who networked sex workers and clients, and who had been sex workers themselves at one point. Peer educators were paid an honorarium for their efforts. Whereas all NGOs used peer educators and a few hired them to work in the offices as regular staff, in 2004–05 the management of peer educators was not regularised. Peer educators felt that their positions were insecure because their honoraria were often late, and they were paid less than was promised in the budgets supplied to funding bodies (for a similar critique in India, see Dandona *et al.* 2005).[5]

Despite the fact that peer education was not regularised and salaries were often late, the power within the relationship was not just with the NGOs (who gained from having peer educators as cheap recruiters). Sex workers also used the discourses of HIV prevention for their own interests: by using peer education for social mobilisation and claiming a new, more positive identity and an alternative income. Peer education has enabled mobilisations of sex workers elsewhere in India (Gooptu 2000), but in Chennai the organisation of sex workers is progressing much more slowly. A peer educators' collective, Indira Female Peer Educators' Collective (IFPEC), has, nevertheless, started from these experiences.

In an IFPEC meeting organised by one of the NGOs, sex workers had the chance to go to the microphone and talk about their experiences. Komala said, "Our parents gave us a name but the police and others have spoiled it for calling us by dirty names and as prostitutes. But now we should be proud for our name is now "peer educator"'' (field notes: 25 October 2004). Rajitham reiterated, 'We are peer educators. We should be proud of ourselves and the work we do. We can't know how many people we have helped but I know that I have changed many lives' (field notes: 25 October 2004).

The above quotes should be read carefully: the meeting was organised by an NGO, and the context was such that the women might have felt pressured to say things that were aligned with the official HIV discourse. Nonetheless, several women expressed their pride at being peer educators and helping others. The status of 'peer educator' was presented as upwards social mobility, a respectable alternative to the demeaning role of a sex worker. These, and other examples, suggest that HIV prevention had the support of (most) peer educators.

In an interview at her house Maya told me about being a peer educator and what she does:

> To take care of my children's needs and other I became a CSW [com-

mercial sex worker] but now that they are older if they come to know what I do, they would not understand. For that reason I am working in an office as a peer educator. I have become a pioneer in educating the CSW by advising them on condoms, HIV and AIDS. I try to change their mind on an alternative income. Now, I am victorious over the problems in my house, in the office and also outside. I am also a leader in the sex workers' network. Like this, women should be able to overcome all the challenges. You can take me as an example ...
(Interview transcript: p. 2, lines 28–42, 20 February 2005)

Maya's account suggests that since becoming a peer educator she has also been able to overcome problems in her private life and these claims could be read as 'empowerment' (for analyses of sex work, HIV prevention and empowerment in Calcutta, see Cornish 2006; Gooptu 2000). Nonetheless, within the role of a peer educator there were challenges related to the stigma that was associated with sex work and HIV.

Some sex workers did not want to be associated with the peer educators because peer educators had to give away their identity shamelessly in public – to 'come out' as an ex-sex worker, and, potentially, as a current one. Many sex workers I spoke to felt that everybody seen with the peer educators would also be identified with sex work, and this would reveal their status as a sex worker to those from whom they wanted to conceal it. Sindhamani complained that sometimes when she educated other women about condom use and STDs, they scolded her by saying, 'Why are you telling all this, who do you think we are?!' (field notes: 16 February 2005) These women were uninterested in 'the message', refusing to listen because of the imputation of impropriety of being a woman who needed this information. But the peer educators were not given an opportunity to brainstorm or learn how other peer educators managed to deal with this kind of response: they were simply told 'go and do it again'. Overall, the HIV-driven aims and projects failed to address the problem of stigma on sex work/peer education.

In the same meeting, the police were also mentioned as a problem: many sex workers and peer educators believed that the police can arrest a person for carrying condoms. Peer educators in Chennai always carried their staff membership card with them, to show the police if they were challenged. Neela, an 'MSM' friend, distributed condoms in common cruising spots after spending the whole day at the office, and was frequently pulled in by the police for doing so. She said, however, that showing the staff card and claiming to be a peer educator and distributing condoms for an NGO did not necessarily protect one from getting bullied, whacked with a *lathi* (a bamboo stick) or taken to the police station.

Peer education has offered an opportunity for alternative employment, positive identity and chances for collective organisation, but not without problems. Until wider social inequalities and exclusion are addressed, the role of a peer educator remains problematic, potentially exposing one to violence. As a global practice, peer education provides a good example of how a ubiquitous model of HIV prevention does not suit all contexts but requires careful local modification.

Using the rhetoric of HIV

NGOs used the rhetoric of HIV prevention to promote the stability of their projects. The following examples show poignantly how NGOs performed HIV prevention and how the women reproduced the rhetoric of the NGOs. Telling a certain story maintained funding and sex workers were integral to this process:

> Yesterday in one of the NGOs it turned out that their 3-year project funding is coming to an end and they are undergoing an audit to see how they had done and if the project will be continued. In a peer educators' meeting women revised under the instructions of the field workers the HIV/STD message – names of STDs, symptoms and prevention, HIV and how they differ, what was the difference between HIV and AIDS, where to get treatment, etc. A few knew the answers fluently, while others didn't remember anything. I wondered if in 3 years, if this was the outcome? – a handful of women who have the closest relationships with the NGO recite shorthands meant to convince the funders.
>
> (Field notes: 3 April 2005)

On another occasion I was present at a funders' review visit:

> Sounds of drumming, pipes and trampling of hooves echoed in the air. Two white horses escorted a jeep to the entry of the office. The band played a fanfare. The guests stepped out and someone made blessings with burning camphor to them. They were two white American women, who were sweating immensely. Someone applied *kumkumum* on their foreheads and they got jasmine garlands around their necks. Needless to say, this was not a usual treatment of usual visitors – they were special.
>   Downstairs, the NGO leader gave a PowerPoint presentation about the project and its activities. Upstairs a project co-ordinator from the funding body prepared the women. He asked them questions of their role as peer educators, what they did and what they knew of STDs. The women had been told to say that they were sex workers in the

area although it was obvious to anyone who knew them that they were not. They lived in the northwest of Chennai, 60 kilometres north of where we were. These women were a core group of peer educators that get taken around because they have learned the rhetoric of the funding bodies. Souresh, a staff member, had to pretend that he was a sex worker although he is not. The staff do not really know who the sex workers are who operate in the area, if there are any, the staff have no resources and means to visit the field. 'They simply fill in the files to look like something is going on' Souresh told me.

The guests came upstairs and were made to sit on plastic chairs while the 'community members' sat on the floor. The guests asked about the peer educator's role, the sex workers' network, the children, the use of condoms. The sex workers told that all sex workers are older women between the ages of 30-50 and that the youngest sex workers they had been able to find were at least above 20. The women assured the guests that condom use was 100 per cent but maybe some new women, who don't know of condoms, might sometimes not use them and get diseases. Of their network they said that they had started to save money since the establishing of the network whereas before they used to spend their money on alcohol. 'Saving gives hope and prevents daughters from getting into the business,' they explained. Guests asked about the female condom, whether to promote it or not. Women responded with enthusiasm, it would be good to promote. Guests asked if the sex workers used condoms twice and women denied vehemently.

(Field notes: 13 October 2004)

Examples like the two above show how sex workers were groomed to give certain impressions and particular answers. First, although many women I met were between the ages of 30 and 50, and while the average age of sex workers that I interviewed was in the early thirties, I met young and minor sex workers who were not in the given age group. Second, the female condom was not available in the Indian market during my fieldwork and thus it was unlikely that many of the women had even heard of it.[6] Third, arguing that, apart for some new sex workers, everybody uses condoms is untrue, as I came to find out.

The answers that the women were able to give, that they were trained for, and which seemed reasonable enough in the context, supported the agenda of the NGO and resonated with the HIV rhetoric. In reciting the rhetoric they maintained the image that project aims were being met and reiterated the government position that HIV was a biomedical problem. The answers aimed at convincing the funding bodies of the efficacy of the actions of the NGO, rather than actually enabling the voices of sex workers to be heard.

The financial interest of the NGOs involved significant amounts of agency and my observation is that in this process the NGOs were not 'innocent' or at the mercy of the economic industry of international aid.

From the viewpoints of the sex workers, the problem of the dominant rhetoric of HIV is that the sex workers' own arguments remained silent. Talking to me outside the NGO context, sex-working women addressed wider structural problems they were facing and raised issues related to stigma, their position vis-à-vis clients, the power gap between men and women, poverty, lack of employment options, and rape. Enabling these voices might have generated discussion on the real problem of HIV prevention: structural inequalities and a lack of general awareness about condom use. What is problematic here is that the dominant rhetoric is disconnected from the lived experiences of the sex workers.

While the official rhetoric was removed from the lived experiences of the sex workers and aimed at proving the efficacy of the NGO, women nonetheless used the NGOs for their financial survival. The process of using the HIV discourse with interest in resources in mind was a strategic process by both parties involved – the NGOs *and* the sex workers. Sex workers were not simply 'victims' of this relationship between NGOs and the multinational funding bodies. In the process of HIV prevention, the sex workers and peer educators were responding to incentives, to which we will now turn.

Incentives and quotas in HIV prevention

All but one of the NGOs attracted sex workers by using incentives to fill their quotas of people taught about condoms and STDs. Staff in the exceptional NGO argued that the incentives offered by other NGOs had had a dramatic effect on the success of their own programme. They felt that their project had not flourished in Chennai (while projects elsewhere in Tamil Nadu had) because so many competing organisations paid the women, and the women were unable to see 'politically' beyond their everyday needs.

For example, I met a woman in a sex workers' annual meeting, and visited her the next day in a semi-slum area. At the second meeting she denied she was a sex worker, saying she had been invited by someone in her area who then got an incentive for attracting a new recruit. The woman told me: 'I didn't know what the meeting was all about. I wasn't listening to the message but just chatted away with other people. I got the *sari* [the incentive for participating] and then came home' (field notes: 1 April 2005). Here is a practical example of how both the agent and the woman used the meeting for their gain: the agent who brought the woman to the meeting gained a small incentive (a common mobilisation incentive was Rs. 10 = £0.125) and the woman got the *sari*.

Each year, all the NGOs set themselves target quotas, such as how many sex workers would be taught about details of STD symptoms, how many new sex workers would be introduced to the NGO and how many would be taken for HIV tests. When new grants were negotiated, the NGOs felt pressured to show that they were achieving their goals, that they were being efficient and that the money they received is not being used wrongly or mismanaged. The funding bodies review the efficacy of the projects annually: the statistics of people contacted by the projects are key indicators. Peer educators use their contacts in the field to bring eligible people to the networks of the projects. Because the number of sex workers willing to be identified is limited, the aim of having to provide *new* women forces the peer educators to find any women who are willing to come. For example, Ishwari was at a hospital clinic where she had been brought for a HIV test by a peer educator. Later it became clear that she was not a 'new' sex worker, but a peer educator of another NGO. The day we met at the hospital the other peer educator had needed to fill her weekly quota so Ishwari had agreed to go for the test.

The limited number of sex workers and the pressures of the NGOs to show their efficiency usually meant that any new women in NGOs were women who were new to a particular *organisation* rather than women who were newly identified entrants into *sex work*. The problem with incentive-led quotas is that peer educators try to make up the numbers rather than actively seeking to raise qualitative awareness among the sex workers about HIV (in 1996 a similar critique from HIV prevention in Chennai has been presented by Asthana and Oostvogels). The fact that poor women, sex workers and peer educators still come to NGOs suggests that NGOs serve some purpose for them. While the NGOs were using peer educators and sex workers to meet their goals of fulfilling their quotas and keeping their funding streams coming in, sex workers and peer educators also got financial and social gains from attending.

The same mechanisms by which sex workers are attracted to NGOs apply to generating information about the numbers of sex workers, STDs and HIV cases. Encouraging statistics of the success of HIV prevention are generated by paid participation in the networks of the NGOs, rote-learned symptoms of STDs and condom demonstrations during which no-one touches the condoms. Many, if not most, of the women attending these events were induced to attend – often several times over, for different NGOs – by the hope of financial reward. For example, when Ishwari went for the HIV test, she became a statistic that was fed back to NACO, which ended up in national figures. This finding may indeed indicate a mechanism that led to how and why the estimates of the numbers of HIV-positive people collapsed from 5.7 million in 2006 to 2.5 million in 2007. My critique of HIV prevention is not that the NGOs per se are wilfully misleading NACO and its funders, but the problems involved are created in the global dynamics that underlie HIV prevention.

HIV prevention is not value neutral

While the economic realities define HIV prevention, HIV intervention is also conducted within the discursive context of Chennai. HIV prevention is not value neutral but rooted in certain assumptions about gender, sexuality and cultural values of what is appropriate: in Chennai, these valorise the purity of women and restrict women's sexuality. These attitudes and ideas were reflected in the relationships between sex workers and NGO staff. Mostly the relationships were cordial and polite on the surface, but there were many interpersonal tensions underneath. When I interviewed the NGO staff privately, for example, they sometimes gave opinions about the women that were against the more politically correct view publicly promoted by the NGOs, but reflected these cultural norms. In these subtle, but nonetheless important, ways the cultural stigma on sex work affected the NGO staff.

The following example is from my field notes, in an interview with three female fieldworkers (FWs) and a fourth person who translated.

> I asked the fieldworkers how they prepared themselves for meeting the sex workers and how they felt about meeting them. They described that when they meet the sex workers they introduce themselves and the NGO they represent. Discussions on health and the family were used as ice-breakers. The FWs explained telling the sex workers that they had this account to fill and funds that they needed. They offered medical camps, and drew attention to the health benefits of the project. At this point Diya, who was translating, interrupted: 'That is what Swarna-madam [project leader] told you to say, but what did you really feel?' The fieldworkers cleared their throats and explained: Initially they had fear about talking to people who have sex with many people but then also felt compassion and sympathy – 'I am also a woman so I want to help'. They also expressed anger: 'Why they went for sex, why do they want so much money, they could get another job?'
>
> (Field notes: 7 April 2005)

The above quote is a great example of the use of incentives as well as a reflection of the feelings experienced by many of those NGO staff members who did not have a sex-working background. A prominent opinion amongst the usually middle-class women staff was discomfort, pity and judgement. Despite many staff members' background in social work or psychology, due to the general social segregation, lack of interaction and even lack of knowledge of other groups in society, many staff members were shocked by the poverty and abjection of these people. When two NGO staff members, Padma and Monica, went to distribute food for HIV-affected people, they came back sad and terrified. Another example is Stacy, a Christian social worker working in one of the NGOs, who told me that she thinks that what sex workers do is wrong and bad, and that every time she goes for fieldwork she tells them to come out of the business. These examples suggest that some staff members found it difficult to accept what the sex workers did or to understand why they did what they did.

What we can see in the above examples is that the discourses of women's sexuality that sanction women's sexual behaviour, and upper-caste norms of sexuality in general, inform how sex workers are seen and thus how HIV prevention is conducted in the field. Underlying the practices of NGOs and the initial attitudes of NGO staff are attitudes towards sex workers that are similar to those present in the society in general – ones that demonise and/ or victimise sex workers. The norms and values regarding how women's honour is tied inexorably into family honour, and restrictive ideas about women's sexual behaviour according to upper-class norms, by which sex workers are seen as immoral, and such values, were also reflected in the staff members' opinions. Another excerpt from my field notes reflects these attitudes poignantly:

> An external advisor from a funding body led a meeting in one of the NGOs. The advisor told the women a story of how morally superior Tamil culture is and told as an example of a folk story about a loving couple who ran away to be together, and only when she was bitten by snake in the forest, he held her hand for the first time. 'The relationship between a woman and a man is holy,' he said. What do the sex workers think about these middle class values, I wondered? I could see from Komala's [one of the peer educators] face that she was pissed off.
>
> (Field notes: 30 May 2005)

HIV prevention guidelines do not take into consideration the power dimensions embedded between those involved in HIV prevention. The examples suggest that NGO staff members were not free from cultural baggage, yet the HIV prevention guidelines ignore these attitudes as if they are irrelevant. The examples also suggest that HIV prevention NGOs did not confront stigma on sex work, but, rather, their everyday practices tended to reproduce it. Notions of purity related to women's sexuality not only complicated interpersonal relationships in the NGOs and led to discomfort for the sex workers and peer educators, but also hindered the HIV prevention agenda more generally.

Insensitivity to gender norms

World Bank and UNAIDS provide guidelines for HIV prevention, against which their loans and other funds are provided. These guidelines suggest that targeting high-risk groups is an efficient way to intervene within the rising numbers of HIV-affected people. In 2004 (NACO 2004: 14) eighty-five per cent of HIV infections were seen to result from heterosexual contact with sex workers, and thus sex workers were regarded as those best able to curb the spread of the infection. Therefore, the essential prevention concern in most HIV prevention literature was whether the female sex workers use condoms consistently. In the context of Chennai this was difficult to estimate from the women's self-reported accounts. Looking at the slowly increasing statistics of HIV awareness among sex workers (see, for example, NACO 2004) it is reasonable to think that they do so *if the men are willing*.

While the general level of accurate knowledge about HIV, and proper use of condoms is difficult to elicit, several authors suggest that it is rather low among men (APAC 2004; Brahme *et al.* 2005; Sivaram *et al.* 2005). When general awareness level is low, and when female sex workers are defined as high risk and harnessed as key actors, the responsibility of initiating condom use ends up falling almost entirely on the sex workers. However, because of moral codes and values of Tamil society that highlight women's chastity, sexual purity and inferiority to men, women are in a difficult position in terms of negotiating condom use. Manuraj, an NGO project leader, argued that the idea that women are able to initiate condom use is absurd. Manuraj explained that women are unable to impose anything on men:

> They are women and sex workers and thus seen as sex objects and socially inferior. Also, men have money, which the women do not, and the one who has the money is the boss. Only if male gender norms are changed, social change can happen.
>
> (Field notes: 11 May 2005)

According to Manuraj, the project leader, sex workers cannot realistically increase condom use and thus safe sex behaviour because of their structurally inferior position in all of the social domains involved in transactions around the sale of sex: gender, sexuality, money and power. Manuraj argued that all efforts should be targeted on men because in a patriarchal society like India it is still very much up to the men if condoms are used. Santosh, another project leader, compared the sex workers to chickens trapped in their cages, and unable to run around freely or to be strong. He said that this was due to cultural ideas of how women are subordinate and they are not taught to be assertive: 'Women in weaker positions are taken advantage of and because they do not know their rights they are unable to defend themselves' (field notes: 14 September 2004).

Both the project leaders were pointing out how they saw HIV prevention guidelines: insensitive to the local culture and norms by which men dominate in the areas of gender and sexuality. Manuraj was strongly of the opinion that the reason why HIV interventions fail is due to insensitivity to local norms because of a Western bias in the intervention guidelines defined by UNAIDS, World Bank, APAC, etc. He said that HIV prevention is defined from above according to ideas that are rooted in Western norms, and they cannot be successfully imported into the Indian context, where conceptualisations of gender, the individual and sexuality are different. This inevitably, he thought, leads into a failure to fully realise the potential success of HIV intervention in Chennai.

It is not within the scope of this research to dissect the relationships based on which the HIV prevention guidelines were originally produced, nor to analyse the rhetoric of the Western bias that Manuraj and Santosh alluded to (see Sariola and Simpson 2008). These notions do highlight, however, that making high-risk groups central to the HIV prevention policies while there is a general lack of awareness of HIV is insensitive to the social realities in which high-risk groups operate. On a positive note, these problems have been acknowledged since my fieldwork and the guidelines of HIV prevention published in 2007 (NACO 2007) include the need to recognise the role of clients in successful HIV prevention. Clients, called 'bridge populations', are seen to carry the risk of transmission to the general public, their wives and children. Although this is a promising direction, it does not suggest an effort to educate the masses – generating awareness of the need to use condoms for everybody.

Concluding remarks

While sex workers are central to HIV prevention programmes in India, the implications of this centrality have been inadequately analysed. Furthermore, what exactly happens between global donors and policy-makers, Indian government, NGOs and sex workers, has not been studied. Sex workers are not just puppets in international aid processes: they use the rhetoric and resources of HIV prevention towards meeting their own interests, to help support themselves financially and to renegotiate their lives. The global efforts in HIV prevention offer a powerful discourse to the sex workers in Chennai by providing a common enemy. Peer educators and sex workers use NGOs for mobilisation, and incentives, just as NGOs use sex workers to maintain funding from donors. These findings illustrate how the emergence of HIV and the industry around it have brought a global dimension to the lives of the sex workers in Chennai and India.

The globalised relationships between HIV prevention NGOs and the sex workers are not just positive, however. They are marked by producing and reproducing inequalities for the sex workers. In a context where the existing understanding of women who sell sex is negative, when a global model of HIV prevention unfolds in the field, it stigmatises sex workers further and exposes them to discrimination and potential violence. As stigma on sex work has not been addressed, only those few women who are willing to come out publicly as sex workers are able to benefit from the 'fruits' of sex workers' organisation and financial rewards given by the NGOs.

The existing stigma and the violence against sex workers in the field, and the inconsistencies of international HIV prevention guidelines to the realities of the sex workers have shown how and why HIV prevention in India is problematic. For the sex workers and indeed for curbing HIV it would be more useful to challenge broader social inequalities, question the centrality of sex workers and other high-risk groups to HIV prevention policies, and focus on raising general awareness.

5 Negotiating the problems of selling sex

The existing writings on sex work in India have predominantly focused on two topics: HIV prevention and empowerment and rights of sex workers (see, for example, Asthana and Oostvogels 1996; Blanchard *et al.* 2005; Evans 1998; Evans and Lambert 1997; Gooptu 2000; Jayasree 2004; Nag 2001; O'Neil *et al.* 2004; Pardasani 2005; Rao *et al.* 2003). What exactly goes on between the client and the sex worker, however, has not been studied in any detail. This gap in knowledge is surprising; when sex workers are central to HIV prevention, Indian attempts to shed light on the power dynamics involved in sex-work encounters would contribute to a better understanding of how and why risky situations occur.

This chapter provides an ethnographic description of how sex work is organised in Chennai, beginning by describing the problems that the sex workers described: stigma, health problems, violence and lack of legal support. These examples highlight the lack of rights and recognition that they face as a group in contemporary India. In these conditions the sex workers nonetheless made various attempts to maintain some control over the sex-work encounter, efforts that illustrate their use of agency. From this viewpoint, sex work unfolds as a strategy rather than a trap. The chapter describes how these women attempted to ensure that the sex-work encounter took place in the most private and physically, psychologically and socially safest way possible. The chapter concludes with reflections on these women's experiences in the context of the theoretical debate about sex work as profession or as oppression: I argue that seeing sex work as a dichotomy, as either oppression or profession, is not nuanced enough to understand fully the realities of the situation. Women's negotiations of their difficulties did not stop them from doing sex work but they found ways to maintain safety and privacy – reinforcing again how positive and negative uses of agency co-exist simultaneously in an individual's life.

Stigma

Most accounts of femininity and masculinity in south India suggest that gender roles are very distinct, with very different standards for how men and women are expected to behave. While all women who work outside the home can be seen to challenge the norm of women's reproductive role as devout and demure homemakers, sex workers are further stigmatised because of the sexual nature of their work. As discussed earlier, women are expected to be chaste and reactive when it comes to sex; the prostitute is seen as the opposite of the 'pure woman'. These two stereotypes are still prevalent in south India. In Tamil Nadu, as in India more generally, women are seen as the carriers of the family honour. Their honour and reliability are continuously monitored, as Vera-Sanso (2006) has suggested, and, when women are seen to break those norms, they are judged much more harshly than men by their families and other people. Any woman who is sexually active outside marriage is portrayed as a threat to the social structure. The public image of sex workers is one of loose, immoral, insatiable, greedy and bad women, and their entire identity is reduced into this moralising representation.

Because of the stigma of sex work, the women I interviewed faced many practical difficulties, such as finding housing. They cannot usually afford to buy their own houses, but must live in rented accommodations in more or less run-down areas of Chennai. If their way of earning money becomes public, they are often asked to leave their rented houses. Indeed, one woman had been forced to move eight times during a span of 6 years. Many of the women were afraid that their reputation as sex workers would spoil their children's opportunities – that their children would be bullied, or required to leave school if their mother's status as a sex worker became public knowledge.

In the interviews, I asked women to describe how women in their communities should behave. Their responses included things like: serving their husbands without questions, not talking back, being chaste, asexual, and looking after their families. These are not simply external values but ones that sex workers themselves had internalised. In this way, the stigma on women's impurity and its social consequences is so powerful that the women who were interviewed reinforced and subjected themselves to it. Shame and fear were common emotional responses to sex work. The shame derived from failing to live up to expectations regarding the appropriate behaviour of women. The experience of being labelled, named, rejected, abandoned, exposing their bodies to many men and living in fear made many of these women depressed and tired of living.

I used to be so proud of my heritage and Indian culture. I used to think so highly of Tamil Nadu women 'cos they are supposed to be so chaste people but now I feel so ashamed to even think about all this because I'm doing this ...

(Ponni – interview transcript: p. 2, lines 23–6, 30 May 2005)

Having said that, some women denied caring what others thought of them, and had found ways to negotiate the negative effects of the sigma on their self-identity:

I went and joined at an export company and while I was working there I thought, anyway I came to sex work through force – let me also continue with it. Morning to evening until six I used to work in the export company and go home at ten and in between I earned some money by doing sex work. The people from the export pimped me and took me out so I thought it was easy for me.

(Swasti – interview transcript p. 2, lines 22–6, 20 May 2005)

Swasti went on to describe herself as having an identity as both a sex worker and as a mother and wife. She was quite realistic about her abilities, and said that she does not need to depend on her partner for anything for she could live on her own, making an income just by herself if she needed to. This positive trope, of being able to 'stand on one's own two legs', was a common refrain.

Sex workers challenge the expectation of chastity because they are, by definition, not chaste. Their disadvantaged position as poor women, who were also members of a stigmatised community – seen as always sexually available because of their perceived loose nature – puts them into a position that increased the risks of their work. For example, the women complained that the stigma of sex work made it difficult for them to initiate condom use with their clients, which, in turn, makes them more vulnerable to STDs and HIV – one way (among many) that stigma affects the women's health.

Health

When women have a social role that is seen as lacking any value or rights, it is very hard for them to exert any power, authority or control over the men they are involved with, either as regular partners or clients. In considering the sex workers' overall and sexual health, it should be kept in mind that one line of thought is that sex workers are not intrinsically more at risk of HIV than are any other people with active sex lives (see Alexander 1987, 1996, both quoted in Karnik 2001: 327; Seidel 1993: 176). The problem in Chennai and Tamil Nadu is their inability to use power in the sex-work encounter, coupled with the persistence of HIV epidemic. Despite attempts by NGOs and the government to increase awareness about HIV and condom use, the risk of HIV has not decreased in India. Steinbrook (2007: 1089), for example, suggests that, because the regional differences in quality of data and facilities make estimates hard to rely on, the best one can say is that the rate of increase of HIV prevalence is slowing down. Despite these problems only two of the women I interviewed told me they were HIV positive, and other, statistical, estimates support this picture: according to APAC, in Tamil Nadu, 9.5 per cent of sex workers are HIV positive (APAC 2005b). According to the same study fifty-six per cent of sex workers had at the time of study at least one sexually transmitted disease (STD) (APAC 2005b). Overall, as argued earlier, given the Tamil gender norms and power dynamics, condom use is not something any women can dictate; it is still very much up to the clients whether or not condoms are used.

In the UK, research has explored the tactics of sex workers to encourage condom use among their clients. For example, writing of sex work in Glasgow, Cusick (1998) outlined five contexts or reasons why condoms were not used and suggested that while sex workers were convinced about the desirability of condom use, in certain situations they were not used. These included: when having sex with a regular client; when having sex with a client who has become a partner; when there was an urgent need to earn money; when faced with a violent client; and when condoms slipped or broke (Cusick 1998: 137–41). Clients' hesitation about using condoms was negotiated by coaxing them, pleading on behalf of their own and their wives' health, or as a way to protect the sex worker – but also, by walking out of the situation, returning the money, and by discussing the sex acts on offer in advance.

Much of the literature on HIV prevention emphasises on condom usage and measures condom use as a main indicator of the success of HIV prevention programmes. Women in Chennai were eager to convince me that they always used condoms but reported similar situations when condoms were not used. Most sex workers had been in situations where insisting on condom use was strictly limited. Not using condoms because of the threat of violence was common. Rape – solo or gang – was a recurring feature of their lives. For example, Uma and Payal thought they were going to have sex with two men, but instead were met by eight others in the lodge they were taken to, and only one of these men used a condom. Moreover, condom use was waived with regular and romantic partners, sometimes because of love and trust, but also because asking for condoms raises questions about the woman's purity rather than the man's, even if they both had partners outside the relationship:

In my house if I tell him to come [to have sex with me] but use a condom, he will not come, he'll get suspicious that I've been around.
(Vanni – interview transcript: p. 5, lines 45–6, 24 May 2005)

Because of the lack of financial security and concern over their immediate maternal duties such as responsibility of their children, in 2003 sex workers in Calcutta did not always use condoms (Rao *et al.* 2003), which put them at increased risk of infections. Their material needs and responsibilities forced them to place financial concerns (for example, their children's well-being) over their own long-term chances of health and well-being. A particular instance of this occurs when the client offers to pay more to the woman upon her agreeing to have sex without a condom. Rao *et al.* (2003) showed that, in Calcutta, sex workers faced between twenty-one and and thirty-four per cent decline in their earnings if they only have sex with men who use condoms. Bargaining over condoms, however, was never admitted in Chennai.

One of the behaviour changes that the NGOs try to create is for sex workers of to use condoms, and they attempt to teach them how to convince their clients to use them. Women were encouraged to talk to the clients gently, but firmly, and to appeal to them with the risk of pregnancy and consideration of their wives' health. The sex workers were convinced to use condoms by emphasising the risk of becoming pregnant or ill with an STD, the potential loss of income while ill with an STD, and the cost of abortion. From the women's accounts to me, it is difficult to estimate the success of this.

Condom use in itself does not guarantee protection, however. Uma, for example, talked to me about anal sex and disclosed that men use coconut oil as a lubricant to enable penetration of the anus. This is problematic in that oil corrodes condoms and thus increases the risk of HIV being transmitted. Coconut oil is commonly used, for example, for hair and skin, and is available everywhere. Thus, it is likely that coconut oil is a common lubricant in all types of sex. Although I witnessed several events where condoms were advocated by the NGOs, lubricants in general were never mentioned at all – let alone the need to use a water-based and not an oil-based lubricant. Uma continued telling me that men also change between anal and vaginal penetration without washing in between, which is another welcome call for infections.

After women have had about two children, female sterilisation is the normative mode of birth control in Tamil Nadu. As most of the sex workers were married and had children, like others of their age they had undergone sterilisation –'family planning' or 'the operation', as it was commonly known. In this way, pregnancy was not a concern to most of the women.

Minor or unmarried women, however, reported abortions. For example, Vanita had an abortion when she was 15, and Pramila had one during my fieldwork. Only a couple of married women reported having had abortions, and usually they were encouraged during the process to undergo sterilisation. Perhaps if fewer women were sterilised as standard practice, condoms would be taken more seriously. If birth control does not need to be thought of, there is one reason less to think about protection. Nonetheless, the abortions of those women who had not undergone sterilisation show that condoms were not used consistently.

Family planning operations brought out interesting dynamics in the relationships of the sex workers, showing the messiness of the category of sex work and challenging a HIV discourse that does not recognise women's other identities and desires. Prevention was not always the women's major concern. At times, through sex work women met men with whom they wanted to settle down and affirm their relationships by having children. At least two women (Ponni and Ishika) asked if I knew a way to reverse their family planning operation. Ponni wanted to leave her husband and live with her partner and have a child for him. As this shows, the concerns of the women were, at times, very different from those that the NGOs promoted.

Sex workers are at risk of STD transmission not only through clients, but also through their husbands and partners. Adultery was common, as many husbands and partners had other wives or lovers, or simply met up with other sex workers. Condoms were not used at home due to issues of trust. Women are expected to show respect to their husbands, and to obey them, not challenge them by, for example, demanding condom use. Demands to use condoms raise suspicions about women's fidelity, but men's infidelity is socially accepted. Similar results have been reported from Chennai by Go *et al.* (2003: 296), who show that domestic violence is inflicted when gender norms are not met, such as when household chores are not completed, women are not submissive to the husband or parents-in-law, if they refuse sex, or if they are suspected of infidelity.

The stigma concerning sex work was also reflected in how the women were treated in health-care institutions. In general, poor women are treated badly in government facilities (see, for example, Jeffery et al. 2007; Van Hollen 2003). Sex workers seemed to receive additionally dehumanising treatment: government sexual health units in particular were criticised for treating them rudely, abusively or in an arrogant fashion. In this way, stigma, at times, inhibited women from getting proper medical care for their sexual and reproductive concerns.

These women should not be solely seen as sex workers. On top of diseases that are directly related to sex work, they suffered from the diseases of poverty, such as malaria, fever, diabetes, chest pain, gynaecological problems, abortions, miscarriages, stillbirths, etc. These medical conditions frequently prevented the women from working and increased their anxieties about not being able to maintain an income for their family. Ironically, many women were unable to take proper care of their bodies because they could not afford to buy needed medications (for example, insulin for those suffering from diabetes) or to go to a private hospital where they could have received appropriate care. Most of them lived in poor housing conditions without adequate access to fresh clean water, proper toilet and washing facilities, etc., which increased the likelihood of infections and the spread of diseases. But to the common hazards of living near to the breadline in contemporary Chennai, the women's health was also affected by the stigma surrounding sex work and the powerlessness brought by violence or its threat.

Violence

Despite their attempts to negotiate the risks related to sex work, many of the women had been in a situation in which they faced violence. Almost all of the women told a story in which they had been raped or beaten by a client, *rowdy* (a local hooligan) or a policeman, or in which their valuables had been stolen. In one of our meetings, for example, Leena had a bleeding bruise on her head: she told me that, 2 days before, two clients had attacked her when she and her friend had picked them up on the street. The men demanded their jewels and mobile phones, and when Leena refused she was hit on the head with a rod. The women made so much noise that the two men ran off.

Rape was a particularly common experience (see also Sleightholme and Sinha 2002: 85–9; Jayasree 2004, on Calcutta and Kerala, respectively). Twelve of the sex workers said that they had been raped, but rape tends to be under-reported, and the actual number was probably higher. Uma, Payal, Sasika and Sangita said they had been gang-raped, when they had gone with one client to a lodge, but then found other men waiting for them and that they had to have sex with all of them with no extra compensation.

These violations sometimes took place when women were not soliciting or looking for clients. Street-based sex work is often described as being most prone to violence, perhaps because of the public exposure. Jayasree (2004), for example, reports violence against sex workers by *rowdies*, but also by members of the public taking 'justice' into their own hands. Unprotected women in the streets or in places of soliciting, such as bus depots, are immediately suspect. Although sex-working women did not use a dress code that would have made them stand out from other women of their class and caste backgrounds, the violence against them in the streets suggests that some clients and *rowdies* can somehow identify them. Street-based sex workers are seen in public: this undermines their chastity and makes them appear 'available'. Vanni complained that men saw them as objects because of the stigma of prostitution, and, at times, this led to violence. A 'spoiled woman', even if she is not soliciting, is assumed to be available for sex: such women are vulnerable and easy targets. A sex worker's perceived constant sexual availability deems them valueless and some men think they can have sex with them without consent. These perceptions are captured in what Sleightholme and Sinha (2002: 87) describe as the notion that a 'prostitute cannot be raped'.

Violence was not, however, restricted to these women's experiences as sex workers. Many of the women who lived with their husbands or regular partners faced domestic violence and mental and verbal abuse, often related to the consumption of alcohol. Domestic violence has been reported as common in Chennai within slum-dwelling families (Go *et al.* 2003). Busby (2000) suggests that in a fishing village in Kerala, domestic violence is not seen as an act committed by men against women, but rather something that the women are seen as bringing upon themselves. Men react to women's inappropriate behaviour, which leads to quarrels between a couple by drinking, which makes them aggressive. In Chennai, according to sex workers themselves, violent outbursts often resulted when partners suspected them of sex work and of having other partners. Consequently, the women faced threats of violence from all sides: clients, regular partners, and husbands, as well as the police. Due to a general lack of awareness, the women did not know, on the contrary, that the law might potentially protect them.

Law and legal agencies

The Immoral Traffic (Prevention) Act (ITPA 1956), the law that deals with sex work or prostitution in India, is ambiguous to say the least. According to this law, sex work is not illegal; however, the conditions under which sex work can be carried out are so restricted that practically anyone taking money for sex ends up breaking some aspect of the law. The law makes no distinction between voluntary or forced sex, and it does not distinguish between sex work and trafficking. Soliciting is punishable, but giving money for sex to a 'single' woman privately is legal. Forcing someone into sex is illegal. But, as there is no legal difference between the voluntary and forced selling of sex, and 'prostitution' is automatically seen as sexually exploitative, then paying for sex is illegal. The law is very ambiguous on the issue of trafficking: any kind of intermediation is seen as trafficking. A 'pimp' is defined by Indian law as someone who lives off the income of a sex worker, enables sex work to take place or forces a person to work as a sex worker.

Because of a lack of advocacy of sex workers' rights, the women interviewed were completely unaware of the law and its details. But the dubious
status of the law was rarely the subject of discussion in interviews, and the
women almost never said that they 'did not like doing sex work because
of its illegality' or criticised the lack of legal support for them. They did,
however, comment on the police as one of their main problems: they had no
protection from the police arresting and blackmailing them. Because they
were unable to defend themselves from the police and were ignorant of their
rights, they ended up having to pay 'fines' to policemen. The women also
reported demands for free sex by the police, as well as custodial rape. Thus,
the women did not see how the law or the police could offer any solutions
to their problems; in fact, they felt the situation to be quite the opposite.
Although the women did not perceive the stigma, acts of violence and
ostracism that they faced as human rights violations, the examples provided
in this chapter suggest that violations of sex workers' human rights are
common and that sex workers are not able to trust anybody but themselves.

Many of the human rights violations against sex workers in Chennai
are related to broader societal inequalities, such as women's subordinate
position, the taboo of sexuality, caste discrimination and poverty. Rights
to sexuality, healthy working conditions, freedom from violence/coercion/
stigma, (the fear of) HIV, and the condemnation of child prostitution and
trafficking are not specific to sex work, but have particular resonance in
this context and have been defined elsewhere as particular to sex workers'
rights (for example, by Western sex workers, and scholars – see Kempadoo
and Doezema 1998; and by highly educated Indian feminists – see Jayasree
2004; Pardasani 2005). The Chennai sex workers themselves had not (yet?)
adopted a human rights discourse.

Unlike in some other major cities in India, sex workers in Chennai have
not formed themselves into a movement to fight for their rights on a large
scale. NGOs that work with sex workers generally limit themselves to HIV
prevention and health, rather than addressing the social and political aspects
of sex work. However, there were three instances in which the subject of
human rights with relation to sex workers did arise during my fieldwork:
once with a human rights lawyer–activist and twice by NGOs. With the help
of the lawyer and the NGOs, peer educators had initiated an organisation
that aimed at being community based and forwarding the women's interests
beyond HIV, but this was just starting during my time in Chennai.

Simply describing the problems of the sex workers provides a one-
dimensional representation of sex workers as victims. Therefore, how sex
workers negotiated these struggles needs to be given attention in order to
provide a fuller picture. At the beginning of my fieldwork, I was first introduced to the stories of violence and victimisation. Once I started to visit

the women in their homes and came to know them better, I discovered that they had developed various ways of dealing with the hazards of sex work. Although the sex workers were in a very marginal and difficult position – one that seemingly does not leave them much space for struggle – the women had developed means to negotiate the risks they faced. They had carved out small spaces of control and resistance within their oppressive life situations and in particular, they had developed strategies to resist the stigma of sex work and the physical, psychological and social risks related to it (for a similar argument from Australia, see, for example, Brewis and Linstead 2000a,b; and from the UK, for example, Sanders 2005a,b).

Sex work as a strategy

Considering the life situations of sex workers using the conceptual framework of agency gives valuable insights into why and how the women managed sex work in oppressive and stigmatising situations. Following the approach of Saba Mahmood (2005) allows us to see these women actively shaping the prevailing conditions for their own purposes, even if these negotiations were not always liberatory in a feminist sense. The women I interviewed had developed strategies by which they negotiated sex work: they were not just passive victims of class and gender. Despite all of the troubles described above, the women could not be described solely as depressed, poverty-stricken, anxious or pathetic. In other words, being weighed down by their troubles was not their only response to sex work. They experienced pains and sorrows, but also joys and pleasures, similarly to many other women from comparable social and economic backgrounds. They lived everyday lives that gave them meaning beyond their time doing sex work, a meaning that, in some senses, balanced that work. Many of the women, as discussed earlier, commented that, before they turned to sex work for income, they worked in the low-paid jobs that are available for illiterate and/or uneducated women and in which they were sexually harassed. In this context, sex work was a more lucrative option. It was not simply a trap they had fallen into, but a strategy that they used to improve their own lives and the lives of those around them – sometimes for better, sometimes for worse.

For some women, sex work meant easy money and an opportunity to earn. As one woman described it, sex work was a 'back-up option' – she had confidence that, if she needed money to run the family, she could put on her best *sari*, stand at a bus stop and get the money she needed. These are women who negotiate life situations for their own ends, using the means available to them. Some of these strategies have to do with the sex work itself, as a reaction to the oppressive conditions in which they must live, and some of them are strategies by which the women do sex work in a way that is safest to them and their reputation. Modes of negotiating the sex-work contact are aimed at managing the sex-work encounter in particular: negotiating emotions involved in sex work and ensuring the safest possible working conditions, as well as negotiating their lives more broadly; improving their situation financially; and having access to amorous relationships and/or subverting normative gender roles.

There was significant variation in how women operated in sex work in terms of the regularity, mode of practice, and the level of intimacy they developed in their relationships with clients. These variations challenge the notions of 'once a prostitute, always a prostitute' and of a prostitute as someone whose whole identity is related to their mode of making money (i.e. selling sex). The women described sex work as a versatile practice. The regularity of sex work varied during their lives, depending on how much money was needed and how they were able to get clients. Ageing, for example, significantly reduced women's chances to do sex work, but it did not always cause them to stop sex work completely. Often, sex work complemented other jobs held in the informal sector, such as maids, construction workers, and in export factories. How long the women had been in sex work varied from 3 months to several decades. They had been introduced to sex work mostly through other women who were already into sex work, or by a female madam, and, in a few cases, through their husbands or boyfriends.

At the time of my research seventeen out of the fifty-six women reported that they did sex work part time; sex-work status was not disclosed by seventeen women; seven were full-time sex workers; at least six had only regular clients from whom they got money whenever they needed it; six women were pimps, although there were pimps who worked as sex workers as well; and three women said they had stopped doing sex work completely. Three of those who did not disclose their current status said they had been full-time sex workers earlier in their lives; another four were minors or were unmarried who had been pointed out to me as sex workers: I did not interview them further. Mentioning these young women without more sense of their life stories defines them as 'sex workers' without giving them a voice, but it is important to include them because under-age sex work in Chennai is not discussed elsewhere, and because NGOs deny that under-age sex workers exist in Chennai.

According to APAC in 2003, in four major urban cities in Tamil Nadu, sixty-three per cent of the sex workers were working full time, with an average of 17 days per month. On average, they had 2.6 clients a day (APAC 2003: 23). In 2005, APAC found that ninety-six per cent of sex workers lived in cities, and in eight districts in Tamil Nadu, thirty per cent of the women were full-time, and seventy per cent were part-time sex workers

(APAC 2005b: 27). The inconsistency between these two figures and the more complicated, qualitative, nature of my findings is unlikely to reflect a change in sex-work patterns, but rather the difficulty of sampling a marginal group who prefer not to identify themselves openly.

Pick-up points and making contact

One NGO worker described the prevalence of sex work in Chennai to me like this: 'There is no red light district here, the whole city is a red light area' (field notes: 2 August 2004). This picture was reinforced as I got to know sex workers themselves and listened to their accounts. Women operated and picked up clients all over the city. Unlike Calcutta and Mumbai, Chennai does not have a concentrated area where the sex workers operate, but there were still some places that were typically used as pick-up points. Research from Chennai pre-dating my fieldwork suggested that sex workers fall into neat categories according to how they contact clients; for example, 'brothel based', 'home based' or 'street based' (Asthana and Oostvogels 1996). My research suggests that this picture is too neat: I observed that women went wherever work was available, rather than following a single pattern. Thus, even if they worked in one particular way for a period, during their whole time as a sex worker they might have used different ways of earning income, rather than only one. For example, they might start as a sex worker in brothels and later move on to the streets and then finally work from their own house. This shows how uninformative the term 'prostitute' is, signifying a role that is stagnant, and conveying the image of a street-based sex worker, while, in reality, sex work in Chennai is a versatile practice. In 2004–05, sex workers explained several modi operandi to me.

> I joined Lalitha, a field worker of one of the NGOs, on her round to do condom promotion. She asked around some of the little shops around a slum area in the North of Chennai to see if they were interested in selling condoms in their shops. We met Uma there and soon her friend Payal joined us. We went to Uma's house and bought few meals that we shared. Uma's phone rang continuously and she agreed on a meeting at Parry's Corner [a central bus depot. It turned out that the meeting she had agreed on was made through Lalitha's husband who was their middle man. Uma and Payal started to prepare themselves for the clients. Payal changed into a yellow sari, Uma wore a *salwar kameez* (a tunic and loose trousers) and a flashing red bra underneath. Uma also applied make-up, blush and lipstick. Uma was visibly excited, Payal was calm. I asked if they had condoms and Uma said yes but did not

show them. Lalitha, the staff member, said that the clients will bring them.

> (Field notes: 10 March 2005)

Like Uma and Payal, working together was a way that many women used to try to avoid violence from the clients. Some women solicited in places where there were many people, and thus potential clients, despite the potential threat of being publicly identifiable.

> At Vadapazhani bus stop, I stand outside there. That's where everyone, ladies, gents, everyone stands, they wait there to go shooting [acquire part time jobs in films]. Whenever I get it [I go].
>> (Sasika – interview transcript: p. 12, lines 35–6, 13 May 2005)

This particular bus stop is situated near film studios and the above comment suggests that women may solicit for both sex work and for film shootings in at the same time, which emphasises the connection between sex work and the film industry.

In order to protect their reputation, many sex-working women preferred to operate in different neighbourhoods from their own. This was to protect those close to them, especially the reputation of their children. In one of the areas where the sex workers lived, there were criminals who insisted on sex or blackmailed sex workers if the women were not strong enough to resist them. Therefore, the women tried to choose settings that were the least threatening. This varied individually: some women worked only during nights, some solicited at bus stops or on Marina beach, some used highways, etc:

Suwarna: I would see clients on the roads mainly, also at bus stops.
Salla: How much money would they give?
Suwarna: Money? Some would buy me cloth, others shoes. Not more than Rs. 100–200.
> (Interview transcript: p. 2, lines 41–4, 24 May 2005)

> I come out everyday, sometimes I get clients, sometimes I don't. In theatres with two to three persons, I get Rs. 150 or so, sometimes I will get Rs. 300–400 and that's enough for me, I will go home. I go to Udhayam theatre in Ashok Nagar. Sometimes I will stand on the bus stop and someone comes with a scooter and asks me. Then I will take them to Pallawaram lodge and they will take Rs. 200 and I will get Rs. 200 and be back by six [pm].
>> (Swasti – interview transcript: p. 3, lines 1–6, 20 May 2005)

As suggested here by Swasti, another pick-up point was film theatres. Although there are film theatres in Chennai that are specifically known for showing sexually suggestive films, or *'blue films'*, sex was not restricted to these.

Salla: Do you go [do sex work] in the porn theatres?
Neela: It could be anything; I will not bother about it. They [clients] won't bother about it. What they care about is that from their body that should come out fast.[1] If not, they will only harass us more. If they are oversexed, then our job becomes easier.
(Interview transcript: p. 8, lines 36–42, 17 May 2005)

Because contact for sex took place in public places, and as there were no visible external markers to show that a woman was a sex worker, it was unclear exactly how contacts with clients were made. I inquired about this during a visit to an NGO:

I went to visit one of the side offices of one of the NGOs that I used to visit. I knew the social workers there and one of the field workers, Zaima, who was a sex worker. With Zaima, there were two women sitting around killing time. Although I had been meaning just to chat with these women about themselves, the conversation quickly turned to sex work again. I was perplexed about how the women find clients or the clients identify them. Zaima said that they stand on the bus stop but do not take the bus. I still didn't understand: A lot of women use buses, including myself, and I had not seen men approaching women at the bus stop in a very suggestive way at all. Zaima explained that the initiative can be made by the man or by the woman, for example by asking the time. I asked if there was a body language or signing that they used. Zaima showed with her fingers a gesture in which she rubbed her thumb against her index and middle fingers as if she were playing with notes. Another example was to place one's hand next to one's ear clenching the three middle fingers and pointing out with the thumb and the pinkie, resembling holding a phone at one's ear. Women started a play to illustrate how it was done. Zaima was standing on a 'bus stop' and the third woman acted as the guy. Zaima made eye contact with him and he looked back at her in a questioning way. She signalled with her head a hardly visible nod suggesting 'let's go' and turned to go while he followed her. I was still confused by this and as to whether a conversation between a strange man and a woman was always a suggestion to have sex. 'Yes, normally unknown women and men do not talk to each other,' the women explained. 'If someone approaches a woman, she can simply slap him.' I enquired about this from one of the social workers later on. Stacy, a Christian woman with social work training, told me that some men look at women – and apparently the gaze is never neutral – but you are not allowed to look back because it gives an impression of lewdness, unchastity and immorality. Sex workers cannot slap men because 'being sexy' was exactly what they were (after).

(Field notes: 5 November 2004)

The above excerpt suggests that contact is made, not so much through speech or vocalised suggestions but through subtle body language and eye contact. I witnessed this a couple of times when I was travelling alone on public transport. A particularly telling event occurred when I was travelling on a bus alone on my way to my Tamil language class. I was sitting on the women's side (properly dressed in a loose-fitting *salwar kameez* similar to those the female staff in the NGOs wore), facing the front of the bus. On the same side, in the front of the bus next to the driver, there was a row of seats facing inside the bus rather than straight ahead. A man in his thirties stared at me constantly. By this point, I had not learned to be assertive enough to challenge or ignore these gazes, and as the bus shook and jerked on the bumpy road, our eyes met a couple of times. At one point, he shook his head with a questioning lifted eyebrow and simultaneously phrased the word '*Poogalaam-aa?*' with his lips, which translates as 'Shall we go?' Although this does not necessarily show he was trying to buy sex, it suggests that men approach women discreetly: due to norms restricting interaction between men and women, this contact is made as subtly as possible. At bus stops, in film theatres and on the beach, contact is made with as little visible sign as possible, just enough to form an impression of what is being sought and offered. A side-effect of the need for discretion is that it reduces the women's chances to make a proper evaluation of the state and character of the client, as her decision to pick him up or not has to be done on the spot, based on immediate impressions rather than a discussion with the client, which might draw inappropriate attention.

For the same reason – the need for discretion and the inappropriateness of interaction between unfamiliar men and women in general – mobile phones have become an important part of sex work and linking up with clients. Those women who were the poorest and also charged the least (i.e. Rs. 20–30 per intercourse) often did not have mobile phones, but were either saving to buy one or hoping that some client (or me) would buy one for them. The other women had a mobile phone and considered it central to their work. If they worked alone, women used the phone to keep contact with regular clients; if they worked via madams, the madams either gave the sex workers' numbers out to the clients or set up a meeting.

In addition to mobile phones, madams were important for making contacts with clients as discreetly as possible. The madams linked clients and sex workers without the women having to go out and stand about in the public, which, in itself, would raise suspicions. Those women who wanted to work as privately as possible liked to use madams, with the condition that the clients they met were from other neighbourhoods than their own.

> I won't go in the morning … I won't go and stand at bus stops. If someone I know finds me someone, I'll go. Once a week.
> (Faria – interview transcript: p. 13, lines 12–13, 13 May 2005)

Female madams seemed to be far more numerous than middlemen, and they had wide networks among the women interviewed. These madams were often older sex workers who had moved up in the hierarchy when they became too old to make a living by doing sex work themselves. In one of the semi-slum neighbourhoods in Chennai, located near the film studios, the madams that pimped women for sex work also recruited back-up dancers and supporting actors and actresses for the film industry. Middlemen, by contrast, were men who worked near the film theatres (for example, as juice vendors, etc.) or in lodges where sex took place, and who pointed out sex workers to clients and vice versa. These men did not take part in recruiting new women into the trade, unlike the madams. In addition, one of the NGOs that worked with sex workers identified what they called 'mobile sex work' after they discovered a group of sex workers who operated as a group with a car/van. Brokers from resorts outside Chennai called these mobile sex workers when clients asked them about purchasing sex.

In the sex-work literature, pimps, or people who help to make sex-work contacts, are often associated with coercion. A 'pimp' is defined by Indian law as someone who lives off the earnings of a sex worker, enables sex work to take place, or forces someone to work as a sex worker. Madams in Chennai could be seen as pimps using the second definition, as they helped to make contact between the sex worker and clients. This was not, however, seen as threatening or as coercion by the women, rather quite the opposite: madams made contacts with clients possible, and some of the women told me that they would not know how to operate alone or in private. Also, the madams did not use force against them if they did not earn enough or go to work regularly. The women did, however, complain that sometimes the madams took too large a share of their income. In terms of 'trafficking' (or bringing sex workers into the trade), the madams did play a role in recruiting new sex workers: the women who were interviewed commonly said that they entered sex work when they were in a financially dire situation and either they were asking around for work or someone (a madam) saw them struggling and suggested that they 'do this'. In this way, the madams could be seen as taking advantage of another person's financial difficulties, but, ultimately, the choice as to how they responded belonged to the women. What the madams did is illegal under Indian law (ITPA 1956); the madams I interviewed, however, never mentioned any moral qualms about their work. They described themselves just as women who had been forced by circumstances to do what they did.

With the clients

India Today, an Indian news magazine, reported in 2006 that forty-nine per cent of men in India have bought sex. If the statistics are correct, one could assume that there would be enough potential clients for the women to be choosy in arranging contacts. The women I interviewed decided which clients they took, based on their 'gut feeling' of how reliable they might be, as well as their personal beliefs and tastes. Sanders (2005b: Chapters 4 and 5) describes this as a professional 'instinct' that develops through experience.

The Chennaite women chose certain kinds of clients to try to avoid violence and abuse. Most preferred to pick up what they called 'decent-looking' men who were perceived as non-violent and respectful. Sasika described an encounter with a client and implied agency in this contact:

> If I tell you the truth, they come up nicely to us, all scared and shy and ask us to go with them. Whether we go or not is our decision, therefore he is all loving towards us. He'll feed us and only because he begs, we go. The husband is not like that, he'll act all boisterously heedless whether the kids are there or not. He's lived many years with me, he should know better and be more understanding. The kids have been brought up by him, and I'm like I am because of him. Just because he pays the rent he seems to think that it's his right to have me.
> (Interview transcript: p. 8, lines 15–21, 13 May 2005)

There was a linked misconception about HIV and STDs: some of the women believed that decent-looking men are 'in families' and do not have infections. In a study of sex workers in the UK, Sanders (2005b) states that sex workers scrutinised very carefully which clients they allowed into the saunas they worked in. The stereotypically 'decent client' was an upper-class man, clean, smartly dressed and always white – all associations that are linked to behaving well and without violence (Sanders 2005b: 51–71). However, looks can be deceiving, as the reports on violence show.

Violence was not the only consideration the women in Chennai had for their clients – they also chose clients based on their perceived sexual laboriousness. Some women wanted young men and boys because they were seen as eager and did not take much time to come. Some wanted only old men because they were seen as usually happy with just hugging and kissing. Some did not take men who were drunk or on drugs because they were considered more aggressive, had difficulties getting an erection, or took a long time to ejaculate. On the other hand, some took clients who were under the influence of alcohol or drugs because they thought that it was easy to deceive them, and the women could slip a condom on them without them realising it, or give them sex between the thighs. However, for all of them, choosing certain types of clients was an important way of maintaining a sense of control and protecting themselves.

After the contact for sex is made, sex takes place in various places and in various ways: in lodges or cheap hotels, by giving hand jobs in film theatres, in the clients' homes, in the 'brothels', or (if they were at the outskirts of Chennai) in the nearby fields or bushes during the night.

> Some people are calling into the bushes and the forests but I'm not accepting. I will not go the bushes and all, I will only go to the theatre and lodge. Like Leena got hit in the head when she went to the bushes, what if that happens to me, who will know?
>
> (Swasti – interview transcript: p. 5, lines 6–9, 20 May 2005)

Those brothels that I heard people talk about and that I visited were not huge complexes where sex would take place in several rooms to which the girls would be labour bonded, as in the public imagination. I was told by two NGO staff members that Jayalalithaa, the chief minister of Tamil Nadu during my fieldwork, eradicated large brothels in the broader Chennai area during an earlier spell as chief minister. After this, I was also told, sex work had moved further underground, while few brothels survived in, for example, Tiruttani and Mahabalipuram. Tiruttani has a famous Hindu temple and attracts many pilgrims – I also interviewed some *devadasis* there – and Mahabalipuram is a renowned village with Pallava Era temples. These villages were described as having brothels because they attracted many tourists. One woman I interviewed in Tiruttani said that the brothels where she had worked were gruesome places in which women were kept by force. The reduction of the brothels can be seen, in that, apart from this woman, few sex-working women that I interviewed told me about these institutions. According to Ms Angeline, a human rights lawyer, brothels were closed down after a central government order was issued in the early 2000s but there is no strong evidence from elsewhere about this. The brothels that I visited or heard about were general indoor spaces where sex was had: they were either small slum huts or lodges. The owners of the slum huts often, but not always, belonged to older sex workers and madams who allowed the sex workers to use them for a small fee. The two lodges I visited were dirty guest houses, furnished to the bare minimum. The rooms had beds and not much more, but nothing overtly indicated that they were regularly used only for sex work. Yet, it was obvious that the lodge workers I chatted with knew exactly what was going on.

Generally, there was a presumption that the sex provided was vaginal penetrative intercourse. The range of prices varied greatly, from Rs. 20 to Rs. 1,000, depending on the sex worker. The young and light-skinned women were able to get Rs. 1,000, whereas the poorest and most uneducated women charged the lowest fees. The median was Rs. 100–250, and anything over Rs. 500 was very rare. However, while vaginal intercourse was the norm, some women, like Sevati, for example, preferred hand jobs, for which she charged about Rs. 100. For a few women, the price of sex was dependent on what was provided. Neela solicited in front of film theatres and at the beach. A hand job in a film theatre or on the beach was done as 'discreetly as possible' and cost Rs. 50–100, whereas intercourse in a friends' hut was Rs. 300–500 (see interview transcript: p. 7, line 10, 17 May 2005). Women complained that they frequently got clients who did not give the amount of money that was originally agreed. Although it was never explicitly stated, this implies that most of the time the money was exchanged after the sex, rather than before. Only one woman mentioned this, saying that she advises other women to do the money exchange before and not afterwards, suggesting that this is not routine practice.

Maintaining control over clients to ensure physical safety and 'pure sex'

Clients were often called the '*party*' or '*panthi*'. The women I interviewed described their clients, without exception, as men from 'all backgrounds'. This meant that the men were from all castes, social classes and occupational backgrounds, and of all ages and marital statuses. When women were asked why they thought men came to see sex workers, they gave various answers. They said that the men were not getting what they wanted from their wives: i.e. 'impure' modes of sex that wives will not do (for example, oral, anal or group sex). They also said that men go to sex workers when their wives are away in their native places, after delivery or when they are otherwise unavailable or disinterested in sex. These women's own complaints about their husbands' requests for sex while living in small cramped rooms with children could provide another explanation for why men visited sex workers. Moreover, Sevati was of the opinion that clients wanted oral rather than vaginal sex because they were afraid of HIV. In some cases the clients were described as young, unmarried and wanting to explore sex. The women said that when men get drunk they tend to want sex, and if they do not get it from their wives they come to them. They did not, however, explicitly say that men are more sexual or in more need of sexual fulfilment 'by nature'.

When I asked women about sex, they always responded in a roundabout way, and it was never discussed directly in casual interactions. Sex was rarely explicitly spoken about, but was instead referred to as '*adjusting*', '*going*' (to do sex) *or* '*doing*', and the meaning of this was understood from the (lowered, abashed) tone of voice or from the body language. All sex was discussed using English words.[2] Because of the participants' hesitance to be explicit about sex, I probed gently, where possible, to understand the sexual encounters. They described to me their restrictions in terms of what kind of sex they provided and they each had preferences regarding the kind of sex they would offer.

Women described that different relationships with different men involved different expectations, and the level of emotion and intimacy indicated what kind of sex was supposed to take place. For instance, in marital relationships, sex is supposed to be 'pure', while sex workers offer acts that are not appropriate in marriage. The women discussed these practices of sex as 'normal', whereas others were not: vaginal sex was the norm, whereas oral and anal sex were seen as impure and abnormal. The division between 'pure' and 'impure' sex that associates pure sex with vaginal penetration suggests a tacit connection between reproduction and women's role in sex. Sex that is not potentially reproductive is impure.

Practice, however, was different from normative expectations. Women's responses to requests for these sex acts from men varied in terms of which women received them, and from whom. Some women only had pure sex with their husbands, whereas some felt that they could not refuse requests from their husbands because of the power and sexual right of husbands. Some women refused practices that they thought were impure, for instance having oral sex or taking their clothes off. Mostly, they said that they refused to do anything more than 'the normal', which meant vaginal penetration with the men on top. When I asked if they did 'other' things, they often frowned and expressed disgust. Some of them said that they would let the clients touch their breast or genitals if the men paid for it, but that they refused to do anything more themselves. They might also refuse to remove any other clothes than their *sari*, leaving their petticoats and blouses on. Having to remove clothes was, for many of them, a frightening experience and was considered very demeaning. Some women, however, said that because they needed the money, they could not set any limitations on what the clients wanted and that they did anything the men asked for – for example, taking their clothes off, giving oral sex ('mouthing') or anal sex ('back'). These women said they were unable to state any demands – the clients were paying and they had to adjust to anything the men wanted, even if they did not like it or it was painful for them. Some women said that they put up an act to pretend that they liked the clients, and that they talked to them nicely, rubbed their backs or touched their faces lovingly in hopes that they would be more generous and less violent towards them. Other women, however, said that they did not make any contact with the clients and would only lie down. Mercy described how she is with her clients: 'I am just a log lying there' (interview transcript: p. 4, line 14, 2 June 2005).

Adjusting to the clients' wishes and whims was a practical way of managing the sex act in order to avoid any conflict that could lead to violence. It was also a way to manage finances; some women said that if they would not agree to do something (meaning some form of 'inappropriate' sex), they would not get paid. This quote from Ishwari and Kaveri, two sisters, illustrates this and contextualises these concerns in issues of women's chastity and Tamil culture:

Salla: Customers will ask all sorts of questions to adjust with them, how do you feel about that?

Ishwari: I'll adjust and go, she doesn't adjust. They'll ask and she'll say I can't and come away, but I'll do it. And you know [whispers] oral sex? That I'll do, she won't. Not to everyone but with regular customers.

Salla: Why do you refuse that?

Kaveri: I don't like it. [Her sister laughs in the background.] Eh, yuk, disgusting. I won't even do it with the hands.

Salla: Would the men ask you to do other positions than you lying on your back?

Kaveri: I'll only do it lying down.

Ishwari: [whispers] Oral.

Salla: Would you keep all your clothes on whilst doing this?

Ishwari: I'll take off everything.

Kaveri: I take off my sari. So I have on my blouse and in-skirt.

Ishwari: I do it 'foreign style' so I'll do everything [both laugh].

Salla: You don't feel shy doing it the 'foreign style'?

Ishwari: [whispers] I won't get money if I think about being shy. They tell me to take off my clothes.

Salla: Do you watch blue films beforehand?

Kaveri: I haven't seen.

Ishwari: I've seen one or two. In the house on a DVD. You can see them, you know, with the actresses and actors from films …

Kaveri: Is that on the TV?

Ishwari: No! They'll show you personally! If it is put on, Tamil Nadu will stink/reek [laughing].

Salla: Then afterwards how do you feel, in the sense after you met the customer, how would you feel?

Kaveri: The stomach hurts. And legs. Then I've some money for the kids, or to pay off a debt, or to buy some household things. If suddenly the body is unwell then I'm happy to have the Rs. 200 or whatever. We only do it for our kids' sake. If it wasn't for them we'd go somewhere and get our food and get a job. If our husband was OK then why would we be doing this?

(Interview transcript: p. 9, lines 2–25;
p. 10, lines 13–32, 17 June 2005)

The women's ability to control the sexual act was related to their ability to negotiate the encounter – certain practices were preferred over others, which were considered dehumanising. Perhaps due to a lack of a professional discourse of sex work as a set of skills to be learned, women's varying levels of ability to negotiate the sex-work encounter, and the amount of fear involved, meant that some women felt they had to 'adjust' to the men's requests, even if they did not want to. Also, the women perceived that men came to sex workers for those exact reasons, to get 'impure sex', so that these actions were an essential part of the sex-work repertoire and thus not to be denied. Ponni provides an example:

Salla: When you usually go with the client, what do they usually want?

Ponni: Most of them usually do normal sex, only sometimes I will be on top, but some of them ask for oral sex and I have till now never done oral sex. They never compelled because I used to sell very well and they are decent people.

Salla: Did people ever ask for sex in the back [anal sex]?

Ponni: Someone asked but I didn't agree.

Salla: Do you do anything like this with your husband?

Ponni: No.

(Interview transcript: p. 6, lines 14–21, 30 May 2005)

Ponni suggests here that there is an understanding of sexual practices that are considered 'normal', reflecting a common view that certain types of sex are appropriate, whereas others are not. The women's attempts to deny clients impure sex could be related to the Tamil nationalist ideas of purity of women, so that making such claims could be seen as asserting that they were still good women even if they did sex work, because at least the sex they did was 'pure'. Using English terms could also be seen as the women distancing themselves from the act itself – it compartmentalises the 'sex' and the 'self', as did the sex workers in the research carried out by MacKeganey and Barnard (1996) and Brewis and Linstead (2000a). They maintained that they were still good Tamil women, even if they engaged in what was perceived as impure and inappropriate behaviour. The women's interactions and relationships with their clients were not, however, restricted to them negotiating the physical safety and the kind of sex that was had. I now turn to how the relationships with clients were affected by psychological risks and how these were managed.

Psychological strategies of doing sex work

An important way of managing sex work emotionally and physically was through drinking. The women interviewed said they would drink at different points: before soliciting to manage the stress of having to go to work, when with the client to reduce the pain from intercourse, and afterwards to reduce the emotions of shame, guilt and stress related to it.

> Whenever I go to clients I take drinks ... See, I can't be very stubborn and show on my face that I don't like it. So I take drink to be a little more relaxed. I will not remember what happened.
> (Vasumathi – interview transcript: p. 4, lines 22–5, 9 June 2005)

At times, the sex workers met together to drink and talk about their experiences. When they did so, they would tell each other about the clients, sex, violence, give and get advice, air emotions and have a laugh.

> Last week I was unhappy so I went to my friend's place and got some drinks and then smoked. After that I felt that I had drunk enough and the next day I started with my regular jobs again.
> (Maya – interview transcript: p. 12, lines 32–5, 11 May 2005)

There were side-effects to the drinking. Being drunk during sex made the women vulnerable to theft and abuse. They may lose control of their own body, fail to look for signs of sexually transmitted diseases, and lose their edge in negotiating condom use. They end up spending their small income on expensive alcohol. Despite this, most women did not see drinking as a problem – it was seen as an important way to loosen up. Women with children who were old enough to understand that drinking was not appropriate for women told me they tried to drink in such a way that it did not affect their children. This reflected the fact that, normatively, drinking is not allowed for women and it was extremely rare to see women drinking or drunk.

All the strategies described earlier represent individual strategies that the women used to negotiate risks of sex work with clients. Women also supported each other, and there were informal, joint efforts to negotiate sex work.

Networks, organising and NGOs

The women stated that their main sources of support were each other and there was an informal network between them. Many women solicited together, particularly on the streets, and they met up together to talk about their concerns, to share worries and to discuss clients. They were each other's confidantes and helpers. The women in these networks helped each other through rough times by lending money, sharing clients, keeping each other company and sharing information:

Salla: Do you have any friends among the sex workers?
Swasti: Neela. We usually go together. If she gets it, she goes, if the other gets it she goes, we never fight about it.
            (Interview transcript: p. 6, lines 22–4, 20 May 2005)

Salla: In general do you talk about customers between you and your friends?
Uma: Yes, we talk about all that.
Salla: So what sort of things do you say?
Uma: We talk about how they acted, how much they drank. And we'll drink too. It's not like they harass us/give us trouble [without a reason], it depends on how we behave as well. If we say we can't do that and kick up a fuss, then he'll do it roughly. If we are all nice then he won't get angry. We [talking with friends] will say 'oh he's a terrible man he makes it very difficult' we might say. We talk well about the nice ones and badly about the bad ones.
Salla: Do you talk only to Payal or … ?
Uma: No, to other friends as well but Payal and me are very close. We have known each other a long time. All her hardships she'll tell me and all mine, I'll tell her. If she's having a hard day I'll

go and keep her company. We go together visiting clients at the same time.

(Interview transcript: p. 5, line 26;
p. 6, line 6, 11 June 2008)

I teach everyone: don't drink. Drink, say, beer. That helps to keep your body strong. But don't go overboard. Make him drink and sit back without drinking more. And likewise use a condom and always take the money first.

(Sasika – interview transcript: p. 9, lines 40–2, 13 May 2005)

Women in these networks were at times competitive about clients, as those who were pale-skinned, young and voluptuous were the most successful in attracting clients. The women rarely criticised each other when speaking to me, but sometimes they moralised about others if they had involved minors in sex work. The networks were also at times quarrelsome; for instance, on one occasion Neela ended up in a fight with Leena at a bus stop, and she spread rumours about Leena's head injury, saying that Leena was beaten up by her husband, rather than a client. According to Sevati, a third person, Neela spread these rumours because she was jealous of not having a husband herself. The fact that the women talked about each other in interviews (when sometimes I did not know they knew each other) suggests that the network that I had access to was quite tight: if a rumour started in it, it would have reached the other side of town the next day.

Sex-working women's networks in Chennai have been harnessed by NGOs for HIV prevention and for recruiting new women into the NGOs. NGOs not only provide the sex workers with an income, but also there is a chance for social mobilisation, as noted in the discussion on peer education in Chapter 4. In red light areas in Calcutta and Mumbai, sex workers have joined together in political movements and pressure groups, and a similar movement was beginning to take shape in Chennai, albeit with less vigour or enthusiasm. In Chennai, the typical response from the women was that they did not want to be organised in public because they did not want to risk the reputation of their children. This does not sufficiently explain the difference between Chennai and the other (northern) cities, and the answer cannot be reduced to cultural differences between south and north India, particularly when southern women have been suggested to be more autonomous than their northern counterparts (Dyson and Moore 1983; Sundari Ravindran 1999).

It is possible to compare projects that have aimed at empowering sex workers in other locales. For example, results from Cambodia, where empowerment projects were implemented in red light districts, but also in rural and urban settings where there was not a specific sex-work zone, concluded that women in red light districts were keener on organising (Boontinand 2005). This supports the case from India, in that the cities in which the organisation of sex workers has been most successful have been those that contain red light districts. This implies that the shared space of a red light district allows the sex workers to get together and form coherent 'policies' regarding condoms. This is not the case in Chennai, which has no red light district, where women's organisation has been minimal.[3]

From the problems and modes of negotiating sex work, I now return to questions of agency and consider what these findings suggest about the debate over whether selling sex is oppression or profession. How the sex workers entered sex work, what their overall experience of sex work has been, and what they got out of it will be considered in particular.

Oppression or profession?

Women's feelings about doing sex work varied significantly from person to person. The concerns of the women who were interviewed and their thoughts about sex work ranged from worries about reputation of their children, privacy and STDs (including HIV/AIDS) to fears of violence. They tried to negotiate these problems in ways that were personal and aimed at physical, mental and 'social' safety. Because the experiences of sex work were individual, an analysis that would logically conclude that selling sex is either oppression or profession becomes impossible. Recognising that women's experiences of sex work were a personal process illustrates uses of agency. When there was no coercion involved in their entry into sex work, the choice to start using sex for money involved some chance for them to consider the idea (and often the women said they forthrightly rejected it due to moral reasons but then eventually gave into the idea). Their first contacts with sex work were often marked with shock and fright. However, after this point, a wider range of their experiences begins. After starting to work more regularly (although this might have just been once or twice a month), women had varying experiences and feelings about their sex work. This ranged from shame and fear to autonomy and enjoying some aspects of it. Recognising that sex work can be enjoyable is somewhat radical in relation to most of the theorising that surround sex work/prostitution. The enjoyable aspects that were described were: access to sex, boyfriends, getting love, finding a lover who looks after and gives pleasure to them and the ubiquitous financial benefit that was mentioned to compensate the effort. Although many women said things that reinforced Tamil ideals of pure womanhood, for some, sex work was also a kind of freedom whereby they challenged the traditional feminine role and broke free from duties that they did not want, such as living submissively in a relationship as a wife and a mother, and so on.

These diverse experiences and feelings challenge some theoretical characterisations about sex work and prostitution. First, there was no one particular type of reaction to sex work that would support it being categorised within the profession-versus-oppression binary. These women's responses do not reflect either end absolutely, but, instead, include facets of both. Second, the different ways of entering sex work do not necessarily determine how an individual reacted to it. The divide between coming into sex work voluntarily and being forced into it did not map onto 'disempowerment' or distress – those that were trafficked were not necessarily the most disempowered. For example, Swasti, who was trafficked and had been kept in a brothel by force, then continued doing sex work and was very independent and determined. Neela, who started off begging on the streets, was disillusioned that her attempts to have a normal family had failed but she was very proud of having brought up two daughters on her own and providing them with a high level of education in a private English-language school. Ishwari had entered sex work by choice, but hated it, while at the same time she liked the fact that she had sex with her clients, which she was unable to do with her husband. Kuntala, who had entered sex work by her own choice, dreaded doing sex work. All in all, these choices were made by the women but under limited options.

Consequently, to use the oppression–profession dichotomy provides insufficient understanding of the diverse experiences of these women. Trying to see prostitution/sex work as one or the other helps to understand the conceptual underpinnings of the categories themselves, but it does not help in understanding the different experiences people have once they are in sex work. Investigating women's agency in sex work from a broadly Foucauldian notion of agency enables an analysis in which sex workers in Chennai can be seen as actors who, in an oppressive context, negotiate their life with the strategic means available to them. From the wide range of experiences of the women in sex work interviewed in Chennai, it is concluded that, while there are limited options and also elements of coercion involved, these sex workers are not simply victims whose lives are determined by their harsh conditions. These women shaped their own lives with the means at their disposal. In this analysis of agency in sex work, relationships constituted a significant way of negotiating and improving the women's lives and this will be analysed in more depth in Chapter 6.

6 Alternative discourses of sex and sexuality

Salla: Did you feel that there was a difference between having sex with your partner and your clients?

Vasumathi: Whenever I go to a client, I take drinks. With my partner, I don't drink. See, I can't be very stubborn, I can't actually show in my face that I don't like it. So I take drink to be a little more relaxed. I will not remember what happened.

Salla: Do you play any kinds of tricks to amuse the clients, like being more attractive, or making some sounds to arouse the clients?

Vasumathi: No.

Salla: What do you think while you are having sex with them? Or would you not think anything because of the alcohol? How would you manage the act?

Vasumathi: I will always think hoping it will be over soon. It needs to be soon over. I would also think of my son. I'm doing it especially for my son. But I'm not doing it only because of my son, I'm doing it also because of that man. I always used to think, 'how will I get out of this situation?' That sort of thing will be running in my head.

Salla: What about with your partner?

Vasumathi: While he was OK with me, I didn't have a problem but once he made me do this sex work and he was a broker. I didn't have any thought about it. Actually, whenever we did it, he would force me. We were fighting about this. The assistant director [a friend who later became her partner] was there and I was doing so much sex with other men but I didn't have an affair with him. My partner was suspecting me and always saying bad things about him so I felt really angry and bitter. This is one person who has not done anything and why all this? That man actually got me into sex work. So he used to force me into sex sometimes and always after a fight.

Salla: What about in the beginning or with your first husband?
Vasumathi: I used to be happy. I used to have climax.
Salla: Could you initiate sex or is that something only men can do?
Vasumathi: I will not, only he would.
Salla: Would you ... When he initiates and you get into the mood, could you then tell him what you want or you adjust with what he wants?
Vasumathi: Whatever he does, I am satisfied.
Salla: What if he became satisfied before you do, how would you feel about it?
Vasumathi: I used to take it as ordinary, there was no other way.
Salla: Would he ever try to make you climax?
Vasumathi: I didn't know much about sex then, so whatever he did, I accepted.
Salla: What about now? Suppose you have a relationship, like with that director, could you tell him what you want?
Vasumathi: I don't have to tell, he'll do everything that is necessary. I actually don't feel like telling it out.
Salla: Would he worry about whether you like or not?
Vasumathi: He wants to make me happy.
Salla: So does he make an effort to make you happy?
Vasumathi: He will look after me.
Salla: Now, can women be outspoken about issues related to sexuality in a relationship?
Vasumathi: Because even though women have needs within themselves, they will not ask outside because once if they ask the partner either the partner will feel happy, she is asking me, or the other reaction will be that immediately he will be suspicious. For example, if they are in a family, they will think: 'I'm going away for 15 days, during this time is this lady going to have a relationship?' This is my opinion why they [women] might not ask outside.
Salla: Why so much lack of trust between men and women? Why all the suspicion?
Vasumathi: The men ... Because men are actually doing all these things, they are having sex outside and having relationships. Immediately they will think that women are also doing it. It's not the lack of trust between them but men have a guilty conscience. They think women are like that as well. Some women are like that, they are very faithful to their partners but some women will go out also. But mostly the women are not like that, it is the men who go out a lot.

Salla: Do you think women are expected to be more faithful and a good wife but men are not expected to be faithful and a good husband?

Vasumathi: The Indian culture is like that.

(Interview transcript: p. 4, line 22; p. 6, line 17, 9 June 2005)

This extract from an interview with Vasumathi is a poignant account of the issues that surround sexuality and sexual relationships with clients as well as lovers. The women who were part of this research did not simply calculate and manoeuvre the sex-work relationships in their own personal interests for money and safety, for example, but the picture is complicated by issues of pleasure, love and desire. These issues are rarely talked about because – as elsewhere in India – sexuality is a taboo subject, and sex workers were rarely willing to break that taboo with me. The unusually frank excerpt from the interview with Vasumathi suggests neatly the various levels that sexuality operates on, the experiences of sex workers, and what kind of problems there were in researching these. First of all, Vasumathi describes her feelings about having sex with her clients and partners. She tells how she copes with her emotions during sex with clients by thinking of her son and numbing herself with alcohol. She moves on to describing how she experienced having sex with her husband, but how these feelings changed after he coerced her into sex work. But when asked about her experiences with her own sexuality before things went wrong with her husband, her answers become very short and the interview begins to resemble an interrogation. Although she spoke more openly about her sexuality than most of the women I interviewed, she is uncomfortable about elaborating on her sex life. Once the conversation is brought back to a more general level of 'women's sexuality', she starts to elaborate on her answers again. She ties questions of sexuality to wider questions of relationships between men and women and the norms that control women's behaviour, but not men's, suggesting that that is typical of Indian culture. As we talked, she provided examples of sexuality, sexual behaviour and relationships between men and women that break these norms, in that as a woman she was not restricting sex to marriage and reproduction.

Generally, among the normative discourses that shape women's sexuality, there is no acknowledgement of women's sexual pleasure. However, the sexual behaviour of the women I met during this research was far from the dominant ideal: the women were neither asexual nor passive in their sexuality. Depending on the kinds of relationships they were in, women used these relationships to satisfy their financial, emotional and sexual needs. From the analysis of agency in selling sex, it becomes apparent that – contrary to the normative discourses of women's sexuality – these women do have access to a popular discourse of sexual behaviour that challenges the dominant notions of heterosexual, monogamous marital sex.

Taboos against public discussion of sex in India

Sex and sexuality in Indian communities have rarely been discussed in the academic literature on marriage and gender. Sex is associated with marriage, marriage is almost universally described as an absolute norm, and discussions of pre-marital or extramarital sex are rare. What discussion there is has been restricted to heterosexual relationships, reproduction and gender roles (see, for example, Jeffery *et al.* 1989; Trawick 1990), while sexual behaviour, sexual identity and eroticism have been largely ignored.[1] Sexuality and the sexual orientation of men and *hijras* have been recently given more attention (see, for example, Asthana and Oostvogels 2001; Cohen 2005; Kulkarni *et al.* 2004; Reddy 2004; Srivastava 2004; Verma and Lhungdim 2004). Gayatri Reddy (2005a,b) has written excellent ethnographic accounts of *hijras* and MSM in Hyderabad. Female sexuality, however, has not been elaborated on to any significant extent. The most detailed account that has discussed women's sexuality and sexual pleasure has been provided by the autobiographical work of Viramma, a *Dalit* woman from rural Tamil Nadu (Viramma *et al.* 1997). This is, however, a descriptive work, and includes no societal analysis beyond the individual.

The existing literature of women's sexuality in India suggests that sex is largely restricted to monogamous marriage. The literature on sex work and HIV prevention, however, demonstrates that this discourse is not without ruptures; yet there is a gap in academic writing. This gap is, in part at least, due to the general Indian taboos on discussing sexuality openly, and it raises the following questions: How do the sex workers see sexuality? How do they resolve the dilemmas posed by the contrasts between the normative practice of monogamy and women's chastity on the one hand, and their own sale of sex on the other? What kind of an impact does sex itself have on these sex workers' sense of their own sexuality?

One might think that if anyone would be able to talk about sex and sexuality, surely it would be people who are involved in sex as 'a profession'? Studying the sexuality of sex workers proved, however, to be very difficult. It was reasonably easy to elicit some basic details about sex work, such as how sex was conducted with paid partners, and the sex workers answered without much emotion. Talking about gender norms and norms that restrict women's sexuality was rather unproblematic, and some women could dissect the differing norms surrounding women and men. Very few were willing to talk about their own sexuality beyond this: when the questioning came to the woman's personal experiences, the taboos concerning sexuality became more apparent and, in particular, raising the issue of female pleasure generated embarrassment. The questions were answered with giggles, astonishment and, oftentimes, silence. How were these silences around women's sexuality to be interpreted? I will begin this analysis by looking at the discourses that surround women's sexuality and how these women talked about sexuality in general, in order to place their experiences in a broader gendered context.

Discourses around women's sexuality

Sexuality is a complex and complicated subject of analysis because it brings together various concepts – such as pleasure, fantasy, sexual behaviour, orientation, etc. – all of which are culturally specific, and have shifting meanings over an individual's life. In south India, marriage is still an almost universal norm and expectation and, as Busby (2000) suggests (for a Keralite fishing village), men and women become whole and 'complete' through the qualities and practices joined through marriage and, more specifically, reproduction. Several of the women in Chennai – particularly those who had married at a young age – explained that they had no understanding of sex and sexuality before getting married. They did not precisely know what being married entailed beforehand, regardless of differences in their ages or whether they were originally from urban or rural areas. But all the women said that they had had romantic expectations – derived from popular Tamil films – about (falling in) love in marriage.

One such example concerns Ponni, who explained that after her marriage, there was a time when she was happy, and her sexuality was directed towards her husband:

Ponni: When I was young, I was quite pretty and I used think I'd get a good life. Now it has all been spoiled. All my dreams have been shattered.

Salla: What dreams were they?

Ponni: There is no intimacy between us, but when I was young I always dreamed of that, my husband taking me out, going out with a scooter, going shopping, love between us. There is nothing now, we just stay together because of the children. There's nothing.

            (Interview transcript: p. 3, lines 1–7, 30 May 2005)

Marriage was the locus of sexuality: for these women, it was unthinkable to have sex before marriage. For example, some women had had pre-marital affairs, which, in some cases, led to a so-called 'love marriage', but none of these affairs entailed sex. Love marriages in India are still rare, although in this sample several women had married out of 'love' (see Chapter 3 for more details on this). Love marriages are stigmatised, and in-laws and natal families often refused to help when those marriages failed, leading the women to feel that their (financial) isolation was a reason why they entered sex work. Rather than suggesting that women who have had love marriages are somehow more sexually liberated, doing sex work could be more usefully seen as an outcome of what happens when love marriages fail combined with economic pressures.

Infatuation with the husband was seen as part of the life stage of the early years of marriage, particularly before children were old enough to be privy to it. One of the women described this: 'The kids are grown up now so we don't have sex because if the children saw, they'd get ruined, wouldn't they?'(field notes: 28 September 2005) Sexuality, then, was seen as appropriate when women were having children, and it was inappropriate to express an interest in having sex at an older age. Once children were 'grown up' (after the age of 10 years or so), particularly if the family lived in cramped accommodation, women described marriage as a practical, rather passionless institution. Therefore, according to the dominant norms that many women adhered to, sex was part of that early stage of marriage that binds partners together and produces offspring, which confirms the relationship and gives the woman a status as an auspicious married woman, and not something that should concern a couple for very long.

However, ruptures to this narrative exist and the women talked about how sexual pleasure is sought by having affairs – mainly, but not only, on the part of men. Women explained that because sex was difficult in marriages due to lack of space, children, and cultural notions of age and 'pure sex', men used sex workers or had affairs. But, as we shall see, this chapter will also describe how some women also had their own extramarital affairs.

The relationship of sexuality to women's life stages says little about how women's sexuality is constructed and maintained, and to understand this requires an analysis of the discourses that surround sexuality and gender. Such an analysis allows us to see beyond the naturalised 'this is how things are' to what lines of thought maintain and recreate women's positions and, more importantly, how the women perceive them.

Women's honour

It has been argued earlier in Chapters 2 and 5 that a woman's perceived 'purity' is a marker of her honour, and that the honour of the family is dependent on the honour of its women. Honour is constituted and observed through certain types of behaviour and actions, such as pre-marital chastity and monogamy. It cannot be simply gained, but must be performed: it has to be continuously reinforced and re-enacted. Central to a woman's honour is her socially functional role as a mother and the primary caregiver for her family. Added to these definitions are notions of women's purity and respectability in relation to sexuality: an important marker of a woman's purity and respectability is sexual behaviour that is restricted to marriage and to one partner, her husband.

The women acknowledged these norms and also, to the best of their ability and in their particular circumstances, performed them. They expected sex to be related to marriage, and recognised the norm of monogamy. They saw monogamy, women's sexual purity and her perceived chastity as a desirable model:

> If you ask why, just look at the cultural norms Indians follow and have followed for centuries, that of one man to one woman. Abroad they simply view it as a friendship and if they can't go with this man they'll go with that man. It is not like a big stone around their neck, they'll talk frankly. But here it is one man to one woman. If a husband and wife get to know each other well and if the man goes with someone else, then the woman will think what has she got that I haven't? The husband was everything to me but then he has gone off, so you hide your feelings and then what happens? You can't go without it showing outside ... she thinks: when he's going like this why don't we [I] go as well? She might say: it's alright for men, [but] we [I] should remain respectable for the kids' sake, our name will be ruined if we go. All this she keeps inside herself but the situation brings it out of her. How long can she withstand all that? If a husband is good to his wife it's like everything good has been sent to her.
>
> (Muyal – interview transcript: p. 12,
lines 24–35, 24 May 2005)

Muyal suggests here that monogamy is both a valued norm in the culture and an imposition, as she describes it as 'a stone around the neck'. She also notes that men are under less surveillance than women, and that women should hide their feelings of betrayal and stay with their husbands for the sake of their children. Similarly, Vanita describes culturally approved double standards over the control and perception of men's and women's behaviour:

Vanni: Due to our culture and customs, when you have one man for one woman as the norm, and the gods sanction that, so then that's how people behave. Those who have 'wrong' desires, they shame them. If they shame you even for talking to gents

> then if they knew you were going with these men, what would that world look like? Because of these rules and shames, they act very cautiously and carefully.

Bhavaani*: OK, so you are saying like that, one man for one woman. The wives may be like that but how many husbands do you know who abide by that and are honest to their wife?

Vanni: They are like that.

> (Interview transcript: p. 6, lines 9–16, 24 May 2005)

These women used the idea of chastity (*karpu/pattanaye*) to explain what was expected of respectable women. Ponni, for example, said that before she came into sex work, she used to be very proud of her Tamil culture, because, she thought, women were particularly pure and chaste in Tamil Nadu:

Salla: What kind of behaviour is chaste?

Ponni: Women, if you mean chaste, is being with one man. Living through with him whatever happens and bringing up the children in a very good manner. My lover got me a gold ring but my younger boy asked why you are wearing gold and necklace and all. I said, it's only covering cosmetic, it's not real gold. But he said, you wear all this and I can't watch TV? So I thought where will I go, who will give me money? The situation is like that. If the man in the family is good, there's no need for me to go out. I sold the ring to buy the TV for him.

> (Interview transcript: p. 8, line 31; p. 9 line 5, 30 May 2005)

These norms of Tamil women's purity and chastity were meaningful and desirable for the sex workers. They reflected the existing Tamil nationalist discourses of monogamy, heterosexuality and women as self-sacrificing. They reinforced the assumption that chastity and motherhood are central to femininity. When a sex-working woman described herself in ways that characterised her as a 'normal' woman she was avoiding the stigmatised identity of a 'loose' or 'promiscuous' one. But the norms that celebrate and restrict women's honour have a shadow of vulnerability and violence.

The dominant discourse involves the potential for loss of chastity through sexual harassment and rape. If lost, women's honour can hardly ever be retrieved. A woman who has lost her honour and is no longer perceived as chaste is rarely given the benefit of doubt: she is perceived as solely

---

*Research assistant

responsible when sexual norms are transgressed, and she becomes vulnerable to further harassment. The women who are harassed in these ways can
easily enter a cycle of further harassment and increased vulnerability. Such
women were often tacitly blamed for exposing themselves or in some way
encouraging a sexualised attack with their lewd or suggestive behaviour. In
the next extract, two sex-working women discuss how honour is lost and
what is at stake:

Vanni: Men look at women as mere objects and it has only been a
recent transition because the situation has changed.

Muyal: The men don't think of the women they know as his mother,
his sisters, his wife. Instead if he sees a tear in the side [of a
dress] he'll simply stare at it …

Vanni: There'll be troubles at home in the family, his wife can't do sex
work [impure sex] so that's why he goes to another. He doesn't
have a baby so he goes to another girl, and gets married. We
are definitely objects … Only money and pleasure, these have
become all-important and therefore the thinking changes.
'With money anything is possible' becomes the motto, respect,
honour, have all gone, money is all. Those with money no one
will look at their back [past] …

Salla: Is it only sex workers who get harassed and raped by rowdies,
because having lost their reputation they are more vulnerable
to it or do all women experience the harassment?

Muyal: All women, it is not just sex workers. Think of all those
studying at college, they'll be dressed decently, with a pant
and shirt but still they …

Vanni: If the girls go with them the ladies get pregnant, college girls.

Muyal: They are just going to college, and these rowdies they think
'How can we trap them?' They look in each of the autos, and
they look at the lover speaking with her and observe where she
goes, they do this over some days and then they – about four
of them – carry her off … and rape her. So it is not just sex
workers it is all women, even those in families.

Vanni: Some have a pleasure in it but then when the lover has left her
and disgraced her then the thing living in her stomach she can't
take care of so she aborts it and so it goes on.

(Interview transcript: p. 13, line 15;
p. 14, line 22, 24 May 2005)

These discourses around women's honour represent dominant discourses
regarding women's sexuality, femininity and gender roles as reproductive,

monogamous and heterosexual that are, at times, controlled with explicit violence. According to the dominant norm, sexuality should be controlled, directed and restricted to the marriage with the threat of violence, no matter what the man does. In this context, is there scope for women's sexual pleasure?

Lack of a discourse of women's sexual pleasure

When I asked Diya, how she felt about her sexuality, she said, 'I'm the best possible partner for my husband' (field notes: 28 September 2004). Diya's remark, and the examples of Vasumathi and other women quoted earlier, suggest that women's sexuality is seen as a matter of reproduction and pleasing their husbands, where there is no space for women's own sexual, erotic feelings. With the backdrop of violence towards those who transgress the norm of women's purity, it is no wonder that women did not speak to others, including me, about sexual pleasure and, particularly, the possibility of an orgasm. They gave the impression of taking only a passive role in sexual intercourse: they said merely that they are pleased with whatever their partners do. Some of the women also openly said that they did not care for sex. Sexuality, they suggested, was part of a marital or loving relationship, not something that was independently theirs; sexuality was discussed as 'relational'. Sripriya, for example, talked about sex work, clients and sex in marital relationships as follows:

Sripriya: Most clients are married and are in a family. The person they marry should act as they wish, that is, they might want to have sex after they are drunk and have oral sex or other kinds, but it is not possible in the family. They cannot have all their wishes fulfilled by their wives. However, if they come to me then they can have the sex which they wish. So that is not possible in the family however they can fulfil all their wishes with the sex worker …

Salla: Can wives expect the same from their husbands?

Sripriya: Yes … women do expect it, they do think about that. If you ask me, I will expect it but not everyone will expect it depending on their family culture, that is, there will be a mother-in-law and father-in-law and they will have household chores until 10 pm. They will have a sister-in-law. But they will definitely expect this .. But they will not say this to their husbands. [Instead] they will take a lover, [to get] what they could not get from their husbands.

(Interview transcript: p. 11, line 17;
p. 12, line 8, 25 April 2005)

Sripriya's example, and that of Vasumathi at the beginning of this chapter, both suggest that there is no discourse of female sexuality that would allow women to talk about sexual pleasure and their sexuality to their partners or to anybody else. The following conversation with Ponni also illustrates this silence about women's sexuality:

Salla:	Would you ever feel quite satisfied [*santhosham*, jolly] when you had sex with your husband or now with your partner?
Ponni:	[laughs] Before it used to be OK with my husband although it was never that great because our hearts were not tuned, but with this man [new partner] I feel happy.
Salla:	Does your partner consider that you are feeling happy or is he quite selfish?
Ponni:	He will also satisfy me ... I can't lie, whatever I think I tell it out [referring to answering my politically incorrect question, this was obvious in the context].
Salla:	Can you tell your partner what you want or he just does his thing?
Ponni:	I won't tell anything like that. I feel shy [laughs].
Salla:	Why do you feel shy?
Ponni:	I can't explain. There are no words. I don't know how to explain this.

(Interview transcript: p. 7, lines 5–17, 30 May 2005)

Ponni is unusually clear about how she does not have the words to talk about sex and sexual pleasure. She refers to her honesty and her inability to lie when she explains how she is able to give any kind of answer at all. Uma, who is married but has a boyfriend, gives a similar account of women's sexuality – or rather, the lack of a discourse surrounding it – and avoids my very open questions regarding sex:

Uma:	The clients come out [to buy sex] because they've been scolded [by their wives]. So it's just '*chumma*' [just like that, casual]. They go as 'husbands' only with their wives. With us they get what they want, give us money and go ...
Salla:	Who thinks about your happiness?
Uma:	Only Dinesh, that man [her boyfriend].
Salla:	Has he ever satisfied you sexually?
Uma:	Yes.
Salla:	Physically as well? Not only emotionally.

Bhavaani* adds:	Makes a climax come, when you're with him.
Uma:	What does that mean? I've made him happy and he has made me happy too.
Salla:	Would you be able to tell him what you want or you'd just be happy with whatever he does?
Uma:	I won't say anything like that and if I ask he'll take it wrongly. It will reflect badly on me. He's an unmarried man.
Salla:	What if the partner doesn't do the right things? How would they know how to make you happy if you don't tell them?
Uma:	I won't say and he won't say.
Salla:	Why?
Uma:	It's because we are like husband and wife, that's why we don't talk about it.
Salla:	When you and your husband were first married and you were in the first stages of love and all that, at that time were you able to tell your husband what you like and how you'd like him to hold you and touch you, so that it would feel good, or even with him you wouldn't say it?
Uma:	No.
Salla:	Why?
Uma:	We don't, do we? My in-laws and all are there. There are 2 rooms. My sister-in-law still isn't married, so she and my mother-in-law were in one room and us in the other so we didn't talk.
Bhavaani:	Would the noise travel?
Uma:	Yes. Only once the baby was born did we move out.
Salla:	Do you think women are able to talk and tell men? Would they accept it? Are women able to express themselves or do they just have to be quiet?
Uma:	They will tell. If they've been drinking ... Otherwise they are shy. Men do it without any shyness [shame] but women get shy. There are women who say you have to do like this for me, only then will I go ... 'What's your friend like! She's over the top', they'll say. 'She's super company!'

---

*Research assistant

Salla:	So, men actually want the women to climax while they are having intercourse with them.
Uma:	Yes.
Salla:	So, would some women pretend that they had an orgasm while attending to clients if they don't feel like it? Would they act that way?
Uma:	Yes, some do that. Now suppose if they don't get what they want at home there are women who go [to do sex work] to get pleasure. But there are also those who go for money. Say the husband doesn't satisfy you. As soon as he comes home he goes to sleep. Work, home, work, that's all there is to their life. In the same way if the men think their wives just go to work and back home, then work again. Or goes to her mother's house they'll also go with someone else. That's what's happening.

(Interview transcript: p. 8, line 25;
p. 9, line 40, 11 June 2005)

These women were able to indicate that although they do not ask or direct their partners in sex, nevertheless they enjoy what is going on. These examples suggest that women are bound by a discourse that severely limits what they can say, but this does not necessarily mean that they do not feel or act in ways they find difficulty in expressing. The lack of a discourse around female sexuality is the other side of the coin of the discourse according to which women are asexual. When women's sexuality is normatively restricted to reproduction and motherhood and associated with purity, not with desire or erotica, it is hard for them to put their emotional responses to sex into words.

All of the women felt awkward in talking about sex and at times the above interviews seem intrusive and interrogatory. Having said that, the interviews of those women who were happy to talk about sex illustrate that there was a popular understanding of sex that did not limit it solely to a wifely duty. In fact, the women's comments clearly show that they are not sexless or uninterested in sex. Those women who did not avoid the questions regarding sexuality talked about sex while smiling and laughing coyly. The words that were used for sexual pleasure were the English words 'jolly' and 'love' and the Tamil word *santhosham* (happy, pleasure, joy). Graphic or explicit descriptions of sexual behaviour were extremely rare, but, for example, Sevati said to me that she and her boyfriend 'have sex at least five times a day' (field notes: 25 March 2005) and Madhu told me that they will do it every night and 'she loves it' (field notes: 31 May 2005). Thus, in what they said to me the women were sometimes able to subvert the idea of women as passive in their sexuality. Sex in marriages, they acknowledged, was not always satisfying and women (and men) looked for satisfaction from others. The next section will discuss women's relationships further, and suggest that women do 'have sexuality'. Sex-working women made sexual choices and adjusted to sexual relationships, depending on who they were having sex with, how they felt emotionally towards that person, what other relationships they were in and what economic needs they had.

Sex with clients

To only look at how sex workers manage sex with their paid clients would be a simplistic way to analyse sex workers' exchange of resources with sex, and their sexual repertoire in general. The sexual relationships of these sex workers were complex and diverse. These women had husbands, partners and clients, and with all of them they were involved in networks of exchange of money and sex. These men could be divided into several categories. There were husbands who were 'normative marital partners', in unions that were joined by marriage. There were also 'husbands' whom the women had as security and façade, who often had other wives. 'Partners' were men, some of whom were 'illicit' lovers (while the women were still officially married and/or living with a husband), while others were short-term boyfriends. Clients were divided into 'randoms' or regulars. These categories are not fixed, but flexible, and in constant change and under constant evaluation. Random clients can become regulars, who can become partners and husbands, and husbands and partners can leave. Sexuality and sex within these relationships were experienced differently. The women expressed clear choices over their sexual partners, suggesting that their sexual preferences were not passive. While modifying their sexual behaviour with different partners, the women suggested they had an active response to sex-work encounters and sexuality. In these ways, they challenged the idea that they were lacking in power and agency, whether in sex work or the passiveness of women's sexuality in general.

The crucial aspects of these women's relationships with clients, partners and husbands are the levels of affiliation, dependency and emotional reciprocity. While relationships with random clients had the lowest degree of emotional reciprocity and affiliation, regulars provided more emotional reciprocity but not affiliation. Husbands provided a high degree of affiliation but only some provided emotional reciprocity. Some lovers provided affiliation and emotional reciprocity, but if the relationship was illicit, they did not provide affiliation. How are these different kinds of sexual relationships constructed?

Sexual contact with random clients

Most of the sex-work encounters that the sex-working women described fell into the category of 'sex with random clients'. In order to manage these sexual encounters emotionally and sexually, the sex workers used varying strategies. To maintain emotional control over the sex-work encounter, the women controlled the level of intimacy in the relationship. For some women, having sex with a stranger was something they could (metaphorically speaking) shrug off quite easily; but for others, it was experienced as extremely emotionally depressing, demeaning, and troubling. Women would describe this emotional distress in terms of their guilt in acting against social norms regarding women's sexuality and femininity. Sex like this was the most unchaste and inappropriate way to break these norms, and their greatest fear was being found out, and being shamed and ostracised as a result. To manage the encounter, the women restrict their sex-work encounters to areas where they could not be identified, and would find other techniques to distance themselves from the act, using alcohol and hoping it would be over quickly. Clients were treated coldly and in the sex act the woman would be entirely passive.

Some women preferred to take irregular clients to avoid intimacy and to avoid having to see the men again. They wanted to keep their work as far from their 'everyday life' as possible, and not meeting clients again was part of this distancing. This was particularly the case with women who had husbands who lived with them. Kuntala is an example.

Salla: Was there any difference between the clients and your husband?
Kuntala: It was all the same. If he had been alright, if he had been very nice to me, I would have been here [at home] and not gone out. But there was not much difference. I thought there would be something for me [in marriage] but my husband ended up drinking all the money and the money from the sex work I used for my needs. I earned a bit for myself also.
Salla: What about the physical intimacy?
Kuntala: I was very simple with my clients. At least with my husband I think that he is my husband and there is some emotional connection also. With the clients I was like a dead person.
(Interview transcript: p. 4, lines 1–8, 11 May 2005)

Kuntala stopped doing sex work during my fieldwork because she was afraid that her husband would find out, and she wanted to maintain a relationship with him. Other women who, like Kuntala, had strong commitments to their husbands, negotiated the boundaries of what is adultery in a number of ways: by insisting that sex work was done for money and not for pleasure, by keeping the clients at a distance, and by not falling in love or having emotional relationships with clients. As women are socially expected to be monogamous, the women's main source of distress came from breaking that norm. Those who found a way of tolerating doing sex work told me they had got used to having sex with random clients. However, some women preferred more intimate relationships with their clients, again showing that the sex workers' responses to the sexual encounter with the clients were not standardised. Hart and Barnard (2003) have described how sex workers saved the sex that they enjoyed for their personal relationships, keeping these acts completely separate from the paid, distanced act. These Chennaite sex workers did not describe managing their sexuality in this way. This could again be related to the lack of a discourse of women's pleasure.

Regular clients and lovers

The women had different preferences with regard to the level of intimacy that they had with their clients. Some women preferred regular clients because they believed that having regulars increased the respect between the two, reduced the risk of violence, and made the men feel more obliged to look after them. In some cases, the women did not call these men regular clients at all, but rather boyfriends. The concept of a regular client complicates the understandings of sex work because, as it turns out, these clients were not just random guys but men with whom the women had long-term relationships.

Those women with regular clients had between two and five men who visited and supported them. At the beginning of her career as a sex worker, for example, Maya took random clients, but now, after 15 years in sex work, she had only regular clients. When women did not want to institutionalise these relationships with regular clients the men were seen just as regulars, as opposed to boyfriends. Maya explained how she made sure she did not get too involved with these men:

> If you start to love any of the clients they will cheat you and go. That is they will try to get as much from you as possible for that reason I don't love any of the clients. Probably I will give a small place in my heart but I will not fall in love with them. Even if I am in love with someone and if he returns the feelings also I will not love them because whomever I fall in love, we will ultimately separate so I do not fall in love with anyone.
>
> (Interview transcript: p. 15, lines 11–17, 11 May 2005)

In many cases, however, the couple enjoyed quite warm feelings for each other. Maya described her relationship with her regulars in the following terms:

> They respect my feelings and also they are not tough on me because they are very decent and they are in a family. They come to us because they are not getting sex from their wives. Only if I entertain them, they will like me and would come back to me and I will be remembered. So they are not tough on me, we give each other mutual pleasure and we understand each other and they deal with me as humanely as possible.
>
> (Interview transcript: p. 14, lines 21–6, 11 May 2005)

Some of the women (for example, Uma, Kaveri and Ponni) had boyfriends or lovers that they did not live with, whereas others (for example, Bina, Sangita and Sindhu) lived together with partners or were (un)officially married. Relationships with boyfriends were less publicly established, particularly if the relationship was 'illicit' and the woman was still officially married and/or lived with someone else. These men gave the woman money when she needed it and also supported her in other ways (for example, by buying mobile phones or paying for children's school fees). In this way, money was not always immediately related to sex. Because there was a certain level of continuity in the relationship, money continued to flow in for the women, and the men got sex and meals when they wanted them. This relationship resembled that of a concubine or a mistress (these 'kept women' were sometimes called '*keeps*'). In these cases, the women were very smitten about their partners, and money was not necessarily central to their concerns. For example, Sangita, Madhu, and Swasti supported partners who lived with them, rather than the other way around. They explained this to me by saying that women cannot live alone: they had taken these men to live with them to provide the façade of a relationship and security. The next section explores three of these relationships in more detail.

Spectrum of sexual relationships

Ponni started to sell sex 6 months before I met her. Before that, she worked in other jobs for 3 years, but they provided insufficient income for her to cover her family's financial costs. She began sex work on the streets, near a film theatre in Pursawalkam, from where she took her clients to a nearby lodge. Three months before I met her, she met a client with whom she developed a love affair; she then became the mistress of this man, a wholesale distributor, who supported her financially. After this, she did not see anyone else. She was very smitten with him and wanted to reverse her family planning operation to have children with him. 'Basically now I am his mistress and I thank God for that,' she said (interview transcript: p. 5 lines 6–7, 30 May 2005).

Ishwari had a love marriage at the age of 16, and she and her husband had two children. She complained that, from the beginning of their marriage, he refused to have sex with her and he did not have sexual affairs with any other women, either, and that therefore their marriage was not happy. She started doing sex work because her husband had no work. She told me that 'random' clients are just for money, but that she has two regular clients with whom she can enjoy sex in a way not possible with her husband.

Bina was married off by her parents at the age of 13. She has two daughters from this marriage, and a son. By the time her youngest daughter was born, her parents arranged a divorce because her husband was extremely violent. Now, 16 years later, she has had an affair with a young man – an affair that has lasted for 4 years. They have had an unofficial wedding, but one which his family could not recognise because of their perceived unsuitability. There are several reasons why two people are not seen as suitable partners, and in this case it is because of their age difference – it is seen as inappropriate for the woman to be older than the man – and thus they keep their relationship a secret. It is not clear how they met. They are very loving towards each other and she says that he has promised, against all odds, that he will stay with her and return to her if his parents arrange a marriage for him with someone else.

Ponni, Ishwari and Bina are examples of how the spectrum of sexual relationships of women 'in sex work' is fluid, ranging from one-off encounters to concubine relationships. Such examples make it problematic to limit the analysis of sex workers' relationships to random clients, because there is a complex range of activities that involve exchanging sex and money. Not all the relationships between the sex workers and the clients were limited to what stereotypically could be called 'prostitution' (exploitative one-off encounters with unknown men). Some women had consensual long-term relationships with particular men and described having strong emotional feelings for them. And in the intimate relationships, there were emotional engagements, feelings of love, plans to elope or to have children. Consequently, to call these affairs simply 'sex work/prostitution' would be misleading.

What this adds to the existing knowledge of sex workers in India is the notion of sexual pleasure. Sex workers, by the nature of what they do (having sex for money), challenge the existing norms of monogamy. But what is radical about these findings is that these women do not just have sex for money in a strategic way in order to get paid. The concept of sexual pleasure complicates the question: sometimes sexual pleasure was the primary motivation, rather than the money. Considering that sex work takes various forms, some of which cannot easily be seen as 'prostituting', it is problematic to conclude that sex work has predictable, generalisable or homogenous effects on the individual women involved. For these women there was scope for agency to negotiate these encounters to be emotionally reciprocal, as well as to provide financial support.

How can we then understand these varying experiences of sex and sexuality that deviated from the monogamous heteronormative ideal? It is clear that generalisations about the sexuality of all women and men in Tamil Nadu cannot be based on the experiences of the sex workers that I interviewed. However, I argue through these examples that there is another, parallel, demotic discourse of sexuality that deviates from the Tamil ideal of heteronormative monogamous post-marital sexuality.

The demotic discourse of sexuality

Alongside the dominant discourse of women and sexuality, by which sex is restricted to marriage between two consensual partners, and in which women have only a reproductive and a passive, asexual role, there is an alternative discourse. These sex-working women criticised the idea of chastity and suggested that nobody is really chaste. They also rejected any binary opposition between the 'prostitute other' and the 'chaste wife', suggesting that such standards of purity produce unfair criteria by which women are evaluated and judged – by other women as well as by men. These narratives were used to manage their sexually 'non-normative' behaviour and in the interviews the women criticised normative heterosexual monogamy as unrealistic. The alternative, demotic discourse of sexuality, concerns other forms of sexual behaviour, ones that include sexual pleasure. Sex can be fun, exciting, dangerous, and makes unions collapse. Behind the curtains, for a variety of reasons, people have affairs with various people, same sex or gender or different, other than with those to whom they are married.

In the demotic discourse of sexuality, partners are not one, and they are not necessarily joined in union. The demotic discourse recognises that young men often do not control their sexuality, but visit sex workers alone or with friends. It acknowledges that husbands whose wives are away, or who have wives who take restrictive sexual norms seriously and do not agree to 'impure' sex, have other forms of sexual access. And women also have partners and lovers other than their husbands, and they can have sex without the intention of reproducing. The fact that some women I interviewed vehemently denied being sex workers, and that their relationships with their 'boyfriends' resembled concubine and mistress relationships, suggests that it is not just women who have entered sex work who have illicit or extramarital affairs. Although I cannot make any authoritative general claims about women who do not restrict their sexuality according to the dominant discourse, the example of these women suggests that other women, who are not sex workers, are also not bound by these norms. Alongside the discourse of women's passive sexuality, in which women are sometimes taken as not having a sexuality at all, is another discourse, in which women do have sexuality, even if they cannot often find spaces within which to act upon it or the words to talk about it. The women I got to know expressed themselves in ways that were not 'chaste', but rather erotic and suggestive. They made choices that were not in accordance with the prevailing sexual norms and ideas about women's passive sexuality. Some women admitted liking sex, and had partners because they were unable to be sexually satisfied by their husband. While one must obviously be cautious in making wider generalisations about female sexuality based on sex workers, these examples do more than hint at the existence of a demotic sexuality.

Generally, divisions between men and women were seen as strongly linked to biology and reproductive roles (for a similar argument, see Busby 2000). A woman or a man was constituted in part through their relationships with others, and sexual relationships with the opposite sex helped to constitute these basic identities. Heterosexuality was seen as a norm among the sex workers, with few exceptions. However, heterosexuality as normative has been challenged in writings on MSM and *hijras* in India (for example, see Reddy 2005a,b), and, among the women I interviewed, the examples of Mercy, Komala and Zaima challenged it as well. Mercy defined herself openly as a lesbian and had been in a long-term relationship with another woman. She saw herself as a 'man', taking pleasure in dressing up in trousers and shirts, describing herself as vocal and aggressive. Mercy's account suggests that external markers were seen as definers of gender as much as certain behaviour, that 'performance' makes one who one is (see also Busby 2000). Furthermore, Komala and Zaima were frequently teased for their relationship in a way that suggested that their friendship was more than 'platonic'. When asked about this Zaima said that she had bisexual relationships, sometimes with Komala. Her relationships with women had started when her husband demanded to see two women have sex together. She submitted to this because he knew about her sex-work history and she wanted to compensate him for this. She then found same-sex acts quite pleasurable and kept on having affairs with women on her own. 'I'm quite disillusioned about my life,' she said, 'but these occasional lesbian encounters make me happy' (interview transcript: p. 9, line 10, 12 May 2005).

It would be misleading to suggest that the women originally entered sex work in order to have the kind of sex they desired, as this was never articulated. Nonetheless, as suggested in some sex-work literature (see, for example, van Raay 2006 – Australia; Oldenburg 1990 – India), sex work can be a way to have sex that is liberated from patriarchal relationships. At times, for some of the women in this study, sex work turned into an affair, or money was 'made' through boyfriends. Some of the relationships these women had were not 'prostitution', strictly speaking, but rather loving relationships. On one hand, then, the assumption that they were 'sex workers' comes within an environment that heavily restricts women's sexuality, and relationships that do not conform to the normative definition were seen as 'prostituting', as the moral opposite of the auspicious wife. On the other hand, another useful way of understanding why these complexities have become defined as 'sex work', when the women, in fact, had various types of relationships is to reflect back on the HIV discourse.

'Sex work' as an epidemiological concept is misleading

Among the women that I interviewed there were some who did not see themselves as doing sex work but instead had non-normative relationships. How did these women come to be seen as sex workers? Holly Wardlow (2004) argues that the concept of sex work has risen from the sex workers' movement in the West and has found its way into academic language to replace the stigmatising term 'prostitution'. According to Wardlow (2004: 1018) a global term such as 'sex work' is potentially empowering as it normalises what women who sell sex do as 'work.' But it simultaneously has the potential to ignore or categorise other localised meanings for exchanging money and sex under this heading, when the local meanings are actually very different from the 'original' definition of 'sex work' (Wardlow 2004: 1038). This is what is going on in Chennai with the use of the term 'sex work'. 'Sex work' and 'sex worker' are epidemiological terms for members of a high-risk group used in HIV prevention. 'Sex work' was a term used by the NGOs and served as an umbrella term to cover many kinds of relationships. The NGOs involved in HIV prevention require an increasing number of women to show that they are efficient and fulfilling their targets. For women in poverty, working as a peer educator in an HIV prevention project was, at times, a better employment option than working in other unskilled labour jobs (like on construction sites), and those women who were not peer educators enjoyed the benefits of receiving lunch and other incentives, such as *saris*, for coming to various functions arranged by the NGO. In this cultural context, where extramarital affairs are socially sanctioned and can lead to violence against women, and many women struggle with finances, it makes sense that some women should visit NGOs to gain access to money and goods. This chapter has shown that the relationships that the women had were very complex and diverse and not all the women were incontrovertibly sex workers. 'Sex worker' is used as an epidemiological–organisational category, one that bears only a limited and somewhat misleading relationship to the everyday lives of the women who are included in this category by virtue of entering into a relationship with one of the NGOs in question.

7 Conclusion

A long theoretical debate regarding the nature of selling sex has oscillated between what have often been seen as binary alternatives: selling sex as either oppression or profession. In sex-work theorising there is an opposition between the abolitionist school of thought (Barry 1984; Jeffreys 1997; Raymond 1998), according to which prostitution is inherently oppressive, and movements arising from sex workers themselves, who demand the right to earn from sex work without stigma or violence (Pheterson and St James 1989). A third position attempts to understand 'sex work' in particular socio-economic contexts have included the work of Sanders (2005b), Wardlow (2004; 2006) and Zatz (1997), who have suggested that sex work/ prostitution is not a universal experience. Instead, they argue, women (and men) selling sex experience their work according to local norms, and particularly according to the law and the protection that is available to them. This third position, which takes us beyond the oppression/profession binary, points to the need to contextualise sex work carefully in its particular local context, with the backdrop of local norms, ideas and culture, which is what I have done in a particular non-Western context – that of Chennai – and at a particular point in time – the mid-2000s.

In India the public discourse regarding sex worker has predominantly been focused on HIV prevention. Among the exceptions, a particularly good example is Anuja Agrawal's (2007) book; she analyses prostitution amongst the *Bedia* in Rajasthan as a particular caste practice, where their kinship and exchange system includes exchanging sex. But such accounts are rare, the HIV prevention discourse has characterised sex workers as a high risk group, and – as elsewhere in India – HIV prevention in Chennai is dominated by attempts to educate the sex workers in safer sex practices. This focus is reiterated in many academic writings that frame their analyses within the perspective of HIV, and propose sex work merely as an epidemiological category. A sociological analysis of sex work that is not restricted to the epidemiological dimensions of HIV is crucial in order to comprehend the sex workers' own understandings of selling sex and their lives as a whole.

This book was framed to look 'beyond' the HIV prevention discourse as an alternative way of understanding the women who sell sex and their experiences within the context of gender and sexuality. The existing sociological and anthropological literature about women in India discusses gender and sexuality in the context of reproduction, monogamy and heterosexuality. The existence of sex workers highlights those women who do not act according to the dominant normative discourses. Who are these women and why do they sell sex? What is their take on the social norms around sexuality and gender? What can their accounts tell us about women and men in contemporary Indian society? In order to answer these questions and to understand these women's lives, their experiences were analysed from the perspective of agency.

Looking at sex workers as 'agentic' follows from debates in feminist research that try to understand the agency of people in situations in which they have seemingly little power (Abu-Lugodh 1990; Jeffery 1979, 1998; Jeffery and Jeffery 1996; Mahmood 2005; Scott 1985). Agency has been conceptualised in a Foucauldian sense, according to which power is ubiquitous and not absolute. Thus, by definition, agency was not limited to 'resistance' (action that is subversive and liberating), but rather as all action, which can lead to negative and positive outcomes simultaneously. In this way, it has been possible to define agency as self-destructive and exploitative as well as constructive and empowering. I have analysed the experiences of women who sell sex through four ethnographically orientated chapters in order to show how they used agency in this way: how and why they started to sell sex, their relationship with the HIV industry, how they negotiated the risks in the sex-work encounter, and how relationships played a major role in the negotiation of their lives as sex workers as well as women and mothers.

Faced with the taboos around sex and sexuality in India, and lacking other practical means of approach, sex-working women were accessed through local HIV prevention NGOs. While the aim was to analyse the interviews with the sex workers 'beyond' the HIV prevention discourse, it was impossible to avoid it completely: HIV prevention defines the conceptual and policy environments according to which sex workers are seen, but (perhaps more insidiously) it was also a powerful discourse available to the women themselves.

The presence of the HIV industry in the lives of the sex-working women shows how the experiences of the sex workers in Chennai are not limited to a 'locale' but are also defined in the 'global'. HIV prevention is an example of an assemblage (Ong and Collier 2004) in which concepts travel globally.

The ideas and practices of HIV prevention in Chennai are influenced by global actors, such as World Bank, UNAIDS and USAID. In studying the relationships of the HIV prevention NGOs and the sex workers, my findings suggest an interesting local manipulation of the resources. The governance of HIV interventions and of sex work is not established solely in response to local conditions and needs, but takes on the perspectives and interests of these global actors. NGOs operate in the conceptual environment that has been created by the global assemby of NACO, World Bank, UNAIDS, USAID, etc.; therefore, it would be simplistic to argue that the NGOs that work in HIV prevention in Chennai are to blame for the shortcomings I have identified. HIV interventions have become an arena for development work, aid and global economic relations, as well as a fight over resources. NGOs used sex workers to convince funders of their efficacy, the Indian government received loans, and the World Bank officials were able to make the expenditures that legitimise their own positions, as well as to enact the Bank's overall aim of decentralising the state. Although an in-depth analysis of this global assemblage and the relationship between the international donor agencies and NGOs was beyond the scope of this research, my findings suggest opportunities for further research on the policy transfer between all parties, the funding bodies, NACO, NGOs and their users. Rather than being pawns of the rhetoric that was used to maintaining financial flows, sex workers were also able – partially and within constraints – to use NGOs and the HIV discourse strategically.

In the mid-2000s, all of the domains involved in HIV prevention in Chennai used a rhetoric that presented HIV as a medical problem that should be tackled by targeting high-risk groups for HIV prevention programmes, and by stressing condom use. This discourse has served as a common enemy for certain social groups, such as MSM, allowing social mobility and organisation. The sex workers of *Durbar Mahila Sangham* in Calcutta have also organised to advocate for their human rights under this banner. In Chennai, however, human rights were rarely discussed. Sex workers are still seen as objects to be incorporated into HIV prevention, rather than subjects and agents in their own social milieus. Consequently, HIV prevention initiatives in Chennai are laudable but inefficient. The women I interviewed were rarely in a position to negotiate condom use because of their subordination in all aspects of the sex-work transaction. Focussing on high-risk groups can be an effective way to reduce HIV transmission, but only in an environment where there is general awareness of HIV and the need to use condoms. Literature from India repeatedly shows that accurate mass awareness of HIV is rather low (although methodological and infrastructural problems of research need to be taken into account here, as seen in the collapse in the numbers of HIV-positive people that I discussed in Chapter 4), particularly

in the rural areas and among women (APAC 2004; Brahme *et al.* 2005; Pallikavadath *et al.* 2005; Sivaram *et al.* 2005; Steinbrook 2007). In focussing
on HIV, the existing interventions neglect the broader power imbalances
that women in general and sex workers in particular face. These findings
have several policy implications for HIV prevention in Chennai and India.
The findings force us to question the foundations and practices of current
HIV interventions, suggesting that the rigid epidemiological connection
perceived between high-risk groups and others should be re-evaluated. The
health-orientated focus fails to address the power imbalances, created by
patriarchal structures, which affect all women. It is ironic that only a social
analysis that extends beyond the context of HIV brings out problems in
HIV prevention and shows how the failure of HIV prevention is related to
(gender) inequalities in the Indian society. Only by developing interventions
that are orientated towards the general population – and addressing wider
inequalities with regard to gender, sexuality, and economic status – can any
curbing of the disease be achieved.

Analysing sex work beyond HIV prevention and health has raised
inconsistencies in HIV prevention initiatives, highlighting that HIV is not
merely a medical problem and that sex workers are more than just vectors of disease. The HIV and health-oriented viewpoint of the sex workers
(albeit acknowledging that some sex workers use this rhetoric strategically)
is a flat, non-productive representation of their lives. When looking at the
sex-working women's lives in more depth, a much more diverse and complex picture appears. All of the interviews that were conducted contained
an explanation of how each woman had come to sex work. Many women
suggested that their main rationale for starting to sell sex was poverty and
the failure of the patriarchal system – a system that assumes that women are
homemakers and dependent on the financial contribution of men. As these
reasons are exact reflections of those given by other women in Chennai for
their decisions to work (not in sex work) (Vera-Sanso 2006), they can be
seen as a public discursive response to the general upper-class/caste norm
of women not working. These accounts of poverty and lack of employment
for women were, though, not the only reasons the women gave for entering
sex work. Two of the reasons why and how women had entered sex work
offer novel opportunities for further research: the film industry was found
to have prominent links to sex work, and undertaking fieldwork in the film
industry would provide more details on this. Also, I discovered that the
institution of *devadasi* is not extinct in Tamil Nadu, and its contemporary
forms would be fascinating to study further. Reflecting on the reasons for
beginning to sell sex invites us to think of the levels of 'choice' available to
the women. Coercion occurred in some women's sex-work histories, but in
many others, sex work was entirely voluntary and decided on in the context

of the other alternatives available to them, and sex work served as a back-up option that allowed poor women with few other saleable skills to subsist when they needed extra income.

Recognising agency in the selling of sex challenges the earlier feminist paradigm that saw prostitution always as a form of oppression. As Sanders (2005b) argues for the UK, sex workers negotiate client encounters for their benefit and in order to be safe. Sex workers in Chennai operated in ways that were calculated to maintain themselves safe from violence and harassment, and from becoming publicly known as sex workers. Other examples of negotiation included: working together, working in areas other than their own to remain anonymous, choosing clients who seemed like decent 'marital types' (and are thus seen as less likely to have diseases). Some preferred clients who were under the influence of drugs and alcohol (and thus more manageable), whereas others found such clients to be too unpredictable. Many women had 'regulars', who offered a more respectful, and thus safer, relationship.

The findings of this research around relationships and sexuality, which challenge the normative notions about women, provide a fascinating contribution to theorising 'gender' in India. Relationships are an integral part of the social construction of sex work, but they are also a way for the women concerned to negotiate sex work and life. Sex work was a way to live outside the rigid norms of womanhood (for similar findings in Lucknow, see Oldenburg 1990). These findings make the definition of sex work very complicated. Some of the women claimed they were not sex workers, but, in fact, were simply women whose relationships did not fit the stereotypical, rigid idea of women as monogamous housewives. This challenges the dominant ideal of sexual behaviour and suggests a demotic one: a discourse of sexuality that is not confined to monogamous, heteronormative activity. These findings raise questions about women's sexuality and contest the idea that Indian women's sexuality is passive and related entirely to reproduction. Still, it was difficult to study questions around women's sexuality: even sex-working women were bound by the 'silence', or lack of discourse, of women's sexuality. In order to understand the complexities of sexuality, sexual behaviour and how sexuality affects people's (sex-working or not) lives then further research is required. This study has shown that people make decisions in life that are influenced by desire, love and intimacy: sexuality not only defines 'what goes on in bed', but also has an impact on people's choices and identities, leading to roles that are, at times, stigmatising and stigmatised.

While sex work provided an opportunity to subvert rigid gender norms, many women also struggled with, and suffered from, their role in the margins. Normative ideas about chastity, honour and purity marginalise and stigmatise sex workers as the polar opposites of the idealised wives and mothers who are institutionalised in nationalist movements across India. The stigma surrounding sex workers has led to violence against them: such violence has been reported all over India as one of the main problems that sex workers are facing. However, in the reality of India, there are so many modes by which women in general are oppressed that focusing on just the elimination of selling sex to create equality for women would be nonsensical. Rather, the problems that these sex workers face suggest that, like many other women, they are struggling with problems that patriarchal society has created. A short list would include dowry murders; son preference, which leads to female infanticide and feticide; 'Eve teasing' (female sexual harassment); and the feminisation of poverty and domestic violence. Thus, the findings of this research suggest that the lack of education for women, the feminisation of poverty, sex work, violence against women, HIV, and the discourses that demand for women to be submissive are all inter-related. This again highlights the importance of addressing gender inequalities in Indian society and the need for mass awareness in HIV prevention. Only a holistic understanding of the lives of women who sell sex – one that includes their sexuality – can lead to well-functioning policies that harness women's everyday negotiations in order to find solutions to the problems of sex workers in Chennai, and contribute to policies that might improve the lives of all women in India.

This book has aimed to represent the voices of sex workers in a way that creates understanding of their lives, options and opportunities, hoping that such a viewpoint does not victimise them, romanticise their resistance or reinforce negative popular stereotypes. The analysis has explored their actions holistically, acknowledging that a multiplicity of forces co-exist in their lives. Important to consider are the personal experiences and attitudes of the women themselves. The numerous examples presented here suggest the various ways that women who exchange money and sex negotiate the sex-working encounter and their relationships with the NGOs. Women can use power, even when placed in positions in which they traditionally have not been perceived to have it. Even at the margins of society, agency can be uncovered and understood. Understanding this – and how women's actions sometimes led to situations that were oppressive and stigmatised and that at other times were subversive and advantageous – has been a major goal of this book. If I achieve even part of this goal, and can contribute to fewer stigmatising reconceptualisations of these women, I will feel that I have repaid, in some small measure, their hospitality and generosity of spirit for allowing me the privilege of learning about their lives.

Notes

1 Introduction

1 Goffman (1968) defines 'stigma' as a situation of the individual who is disqualified from full social acceptance. In Chennai, selling sex is seen as disrespectful, polluted, pitiful and deviant. Those who do, or are perceived to, sell sex are labelled as 'loose', 'lacking social value' and 'immoral'.

2 Contextualising sex work in Chennai

1 *Devadasis* were a caste of women who performed dance and religious rituals in Hindu temples, which at times included sex with priests and pilgrims, and who were deemed as prostitutes during a social reform in late nineteenth century. The institution was eventually banned but there is evidence that *devadasi* women still exist.

2 See Caplan (1985) on upper-class women in Chennai; Hancock (1999) on orthodox Tamil Brahman women; Jeffery (1979) on upper-class Muslim women; Trawick (1990) on Tamil upper caste women; and Wadley (1980a) on Tamil women in general.

3 Feminist scholars have debated the role and level of agency involved in *purdah*. Jeffery (1979) argued that the women themselves have a role in the maintenance of *purdah* and are not just socialised into this role – not simply pawns of patriarchal gender oppression, but also agents able to see 'beyond themselves'. Women do not take *purdah* without complying, and the younger generation in particular is aware of the limitations that *purdah* and the isolation it causes. This analysis allows more agency for women. Women are not victimized as 'Third World women' but the analysis of agency recognises that women have various amounts of power; for example (depending on their position in the family): the newly married wife, the unmarried daughter, a mother-in-law, widowed grandmother, etc.

4 Impurity of childbirth has also been observed by Van Hollen (2003) in Tamil Nadu and by Jeffery *et al.* (1989) in Uttar Pradesh.

3 Women in sex work

1 This is a reference to venues where sex is had. Some sex workers used particular houses for sex. The house owner, who was not necessarily a sex worker,

got a cut from the earnings. I will describe the social construction of sex work further in Chapter 5.

2 The question of *devadasis* requires further research. The *devadasi* institution was officially abolished in the 1950s. However, from my findings and research from the neighbouring state Karnataka (O'Neil *et al.* 2004), it is apparent that *devadasis* still exist. The women I interviewed suggest that there are two types of *devadasi*. This was also suggested by an NGO leader from another area. There are those who are similar to those *devadasis* from the past – who are typified by caste lineage and who work at the temples – and there are those who have been sacrificed to temples by their parents in ritualistic exchanges (for example, in hoping to cure a fatal disease). These women can stay in their homes rather than moving to the temple, but they are officially married to the gods and cannot thus marry a man.

3 Women's participation in the informal employment sector has been researched by Swaminathan (2004), and she and many others (see, for example, Moghadam 2005) have suggested that the introduction of capitalism in India and elsewhere has feminised poverty in that women represent labour power that gets the worst paid jobs because women tend not to belong to labour unions.

4 CAPACS (www.capacs.org/ngos.htm), retrieved on 21 October 2008; TAI (www.taivhs.org/about.htm), retrieved on 21 October 2008; APAC (www.apacvhs.org/OurPar_NGOs.html), retrieved on 21 October 2008.

5 Following changes in HIV prevention practices since my fieldwork (NACO 2007), the role of community-based organizations has become more prominent in HIV prevention along the lines suggested here.

6 The BBC reported on 17 March 2007 that Tamil Nadu will launch female condoms on a grand scale.

5 Negotiating the problems of selling sex

1 Note the roundabout way of talking about ejaculation. I will discuss how sex was talked about later in this chapter, as well as in Chapter 6.

2 Based on the language used by sex workers in Calcutta, Dell (2005) argues that certain sexual acts are associated with impurity due to the nationalist dichotomy of women's purity – 'sexual' being the polar opposite of 'pure'. Following the logic of trying to construct a positive identity against colonisers, Dell argues that, in this discourse, Indians were constructed as spiritual and pure, whereas all that was considered impure was associated with the colonisers and was discussed using the English words.

3 Cornish (2006: 302) has argued that areas that have a tradition of trade unions can facilitate the organisation of sex workers. This would suggest that because Bengal has a history of trade unions, the idea that sex workers as workers who should form unions is not as odd an idea. In Chennai, the dominant form of organization has been related to Tamil nationalism, which valorises purity of women (for party politics, see, for example, Gorringe 2005; for women's organizations, see Caplan 1985) and thus is less conducive to the organisation of the sex workers.

6 Alternative discourses of sex and sexuality

1 For exceptions, see, for example, Paul Hershman (1974). Also Jeffery and

Jeffery (1996) show that women's songs, sung either after childbirth or at weddings, hint at women's active sexuality in ways that are not admissible in everyday public discussions. John and Nair (1998) edited a book *A Question of Silence: Sexual Economies of Modern India*, but articles in this are either historical analyses or analyse media/literature representations and not based on fieldwork.

Appendix

List of sex workers part of the research

1 Ambuja was in her forties. Her ethnic background is Telegu. She had a love marriage with her husband. Her husband had other wives over the years but they continued to live together and have three children. Ambuja also worked in the film industry. She was a peer educator.
2 Avantika was 33 years old. She was a *devadasi*. She was unmarried but was the second wife of her partner.
3 Bhubamma was about 60 years old. She had two children, one of whom was adopted. Widowed. Bhubamma sold sex for several decades and at the time of research was a pimp. She was one of the leading figures in one of the NGOs and a peer educator.
4 Bina was 32 years old. She went to school till fifth standard. She had an arranged marriage at the age of 12, but her husband was violent and she had a divorce. At the time of my research she had a relationship with a younger man and she said she was not a sex worker. She had two daughters and a son. Peer educator.
5 Chapala was about 25 years old. She married a man who raped her but later separated from him. At the time of my research, Chapala lived with her sister Ishika and they looked after their children together. She had no education, and had been involved in sex work for 3 years, part time. She charged about Rs. 20–30 per client.
6 Diya was 33 years old. She had completed eighth standard at school. Diya was married with two children, but also had partners. She had sold sex for 4 years, part time, and earned about Rs. 4,000 per month. Peer educator.
7 Faria was 34 years old. Faria was from Scheduled Caste background. She had a love marriage at the age of 16 but had been widowed since. She called herself a *keep*, meaning that she was involved with a man who already had wife. She had three children. She worked along highways and earned about Rs. 200 per client, but also attended film shootings to act as a background dancer.

8   Ishika was 29 years old. She had a love marriage with a man who had other wives and, at the time of my research, had two children and lived with them and her sister Chapala. Ishika earned Rs. 20–30 per client.

9   Ishwari was 28 years old. She had a love marriage at the age of 16. She lived with her husband, although she had partners. She had two children with her husband. She had completed tenth standard at school. She is from a Telegu *Naidu* caste background. She had sold sex for 2 years, full time. Ishwari was a peer educator.

10 Jeevitha was in her fifties. She had an arranged marriage at the age of 12, but, at the time of my research, she was single. She had two sons. She said she had been doing sex work 'for decades'.

11 Jaisanthi was about 35. She had been married, but, at the time of my research, she was single. She had one child. She had been doing sex work for 8 years and earned about Rs. 300 per client.

12 Joshita was 27 years old. She had an arranged marriage at the age of 14, and lived with her husband and in-laws at the time of my research. She had three children. She had sold sex for 4 years on a part-time basis. Her sister-in-law Pugazh, and mother-in-law Jeevitha were in sex work as well, and there were rumours about her minor daughter.

13 Jayati was 32 years old. She had completed tenth standard at school. She was married but separated, and, at the time of my research, had a partner. She had two children. She earned about Rs. 10,000 per month from selling sex and ran a gift shop as a façade.

14 Jeevitha was about 50 years old. She was married and lived with her husband, two sons and their wives – she was the mother-in-law of Joshita and Pugazh. She had been to sex work for several decades and acted as a pimp.

15 Kanchi was 37 years old. She had completed fifth standard at school. She was married but lived alone at the time of my research, and was someone's second wife. She has children (but it was unclear to me how many). She had sold sex for 7 years and earned Rs. 50–100 per client. She also sold flower chains on streets and worked as a maid.

16 Kaveri was 28 years old. She was from Telegu *Naidu* caste background. She had an arranged marriage at the age of 14, but, at the time of my research, was single. She had one main partner, sometimes others. She had sold sex for 1.5 years. Ishika's sister.

17 Komala had been married but was since widowed. She lived with her one son. President of the peer educators' association. She was the occasional lover of Zaima.

18 Kuntala was 24 years old. She had completed tenth standard at school. She spoke Telegu as her first language. She had an arranged marriage at the age of 15 and lived with her husband. They had two children

together and looked after a nephew. She had been doing sex work for 5 years but stopped during the time of my fieldwork. Peer educator.

19 Leena was 27 years old. She had completed fifth standard at school. She married at the age of 16 and lived with her husband. They had two children. She had sold sex for 5 years, full-time and earned Rs. 6,500 per month. Leena also worked as a maid.

20 Lavali was 32 years old. She had studied till eighth standard at school. She was married at the age of 18 but had remarried since. She had two children. She had sold sex for 12 years.

21 Mahadevi was 38 years old. She had completed tenth standard at school. She was married with three children. She had spent 5 years in sex work.

22 Manjula was about 50 years old. She was a *devadasi*, unmarried, and lived alone, but had multiple partners. She looked after her sister's four children, whom she had adopted.

23 Maria was 18 years old. She had no schooling. She was unmarried and lived with her family. Her sister was also a sex worker (Sheila).

24 Maya was 35 years old. She had completed twelfth standard at school. She was married at the age of 18 in a love marriage but separated since. At the time of my research she had boyfriends. She had two children. She had been in sex work for 15 years on a part-time basis – her partners gave her money whenever she needed it. Peer educator.

25 Mercy was 25 years old. She was from a Malayali background. She had completed ninth standard at school. She had an arranged marriage, but was widowed, and, at the time of my research, lived alone. She had one child, and had a miscarriage during my fieldwork. She identified herself as a lesbian. She had worked as a sex worker for 5 years, part time, and earned Rs. 1,000 per client. She also worked in the film industry. Peer educator.

26 Muyal was 35 years old. She had completed eighth standard at school. She had a love marriage but at the time of my research she had partners/regulars. She had two children. She also worked in films as a background actress. Peer educator.

27 Madhu was 28 years old. She had not undergone any schooling. Madhu was married at the age of eight to a man much older than her, but separated since and at the time of my research lived with her boyfriend. She had two children who did not live with her. She had sold sex for 9 years, also worked in films, and, occasionally, donated blood for money.

28 Neela was 34 years old. She had completed fifth standard at school. She married at the age of 16 but separated, and since then had consecutive partners, but none of these relationships lasted. Lived with her two

daughters. She had been doing sex work for 12 years and earned about Rs. 200–300 per client. Peer educator.

29   Nidhi was 43 years old. She was a Muslim. She had studied till eighth standard. She was married at the age of 16, but, at the time of my research, lived with her sister and has five children. She was mostly making money through pimping. Peer educator.

30   Nitya was 34 years old. She comes from a *Naidu* caste background. She was married at the age of 13, but, at the time of my research, lived with a partner. Nitya was a full-time sex worker and earned about Rs. 1,000 per week.

31   Payal was 34 years old. She had completed fifth standard at school. She had an arranged marriage, and, at the time of my research, lived with her husband and three children.

32   Ponni was 30 years old. She had finished seventh standard at school. She had had an arranged married at the age of 17. At the time of my research she lived with her husband but also had a boyfriend/partner. She had two children. She had been doing sex work for 6 months, part time, earning Rs. 400 per month.

33   Pooja was married with two children. Peer educator.

34   Pramila was about 20. She was unmarried and had an abortion during the time of my fieldwork.

35   Pratima was about 50 years old. She was married. She ran a savings scheme for the women. We talked about this only in our interview, although I met her regularly in the NGOs.

36   Pugazh was 27 years old. She had a love marriage with a man from a lower caste at the age of 13. They had two children. Her mother-in-law (Jeevitha) and sister-in-law (Joshita) were also sex workers. She took regular customers.

37   Revati was 38 years old. She was unmarried, lived with her partner, and had three children. She had been working in the sex industry since childhood – she was initially trafficked and then continued on her own. Peer educator.

38   Rajitham was 28 years old. She had been married but was widowed, and, at the time of my research, had lovers/partners. She had three children. She had been doing sex work for 5 years, but, at the time of my research, only pimped. She was HIV positive.

39   Sheila was 14 years old. She had no schooling, was unmarried and lived with her family. Her sister was a sex worker (Maria).

40   Sevati was 29 years old. She was single, lived with her sister, and her partner stayed with them at times. She had been doing sex work for 'long', and she worked full time. Peer educator.

41   Sonali was 21 years old. She was unmarried and lived with her sister,

who was a sex worker (Sevati). Whether or not Sonali was a sex worker remained unclear.

42 Sindhamani was in her forties. She was married to a government worker and they had had three children. Her husband died in an accident. She says she was not a sex worker, but she worked as a peer educator.

43 Sasika was 38 years old. She was first married to a relative at the age of 16, but then widowed. She lived with her second husband with whom she had a love marriage. She did sex work on a part-time basis and also worked in the film industry as a supporting actress. She had one daughter who was also a sex worker (Vanita).

44 Sharita was 35 years old. She had completed tenth standard at school. She had two children and lived with them and a boyfriend. She had been involved in sex work for 2 years, part time, and earned Rs. 5,000 per month.

45 Sheelamma was about 50 years old. She came from a land-owning family in Kerala. She had been married but was now divorced and at the time of my research she lived alone. She had five children, who were brought up in a convent and by relatives – she had no contact with them. She had been in sex work for several decades, and was also a pimp. She was a peer educator and central figure in the women's organisation.

46 Sangita was 23 years old. She was a Muslim. She had no schooling. Sangita had, initially, a love marriage but later separated from her husband, and, at the time of my research, had a partner. She has three children. She worked in sex work on a full-time basis and earned about Rs. 2,000 per month.

47 Swasti was 35 years old. She was married at the age of 15 but then divorced, and, at the time of my research, lived with a partner. She had three children. Swasti was initially trafficked but then continued working on her own on a full-time basis, earning about Rs. 1,500 per month. She also worked in an export company and as a peer educator.

48 Sudevi was 35 years old. She had completed fifth standard at school. She was married at the age of 15 and had two children. She had regular clients.

49 Sripriya was 35 years old. She comes from a *Chettiyar* caste and her paternal aunts were *devadasis*. She had an arranged marriage at the age of 16 but then separated from her husband, and, at the time of my research, she lived with her partner. She had two children. She had sold sex for about 10 years, but, at the time of my fieldwork, she had stopped. She was a peer educator.

50 Swarna was 36 years old. She had completed eighth standard at school. She was married to a lover, and had one daughter. She had been in sex

work for 20 years and used to work on a part-time basis, but, during my fieldwork, she had stopped. She was HIV positive.

51 Sindhu was 41 years old. She was married at the age of 15 but then separated from her husband, and, at the time of my research, had a new partner. She had four children, one of whom was disabled and lived in a care home, funded by an NGO. She had been a sex worker for 13 years, but also worked as a maid.

52 Uma was 25 years old. Uma lived with her husband with whom she had love marriage. They had five children out of which only one survived. During my fieldwork she had a tumultuous love affair that led her to pour kerosene over herself. She had been in sex work for 5 years, full-time, and also pimped. Peer educator.

53 Vanita was 17 years old. She had completed fifth standard at school. She was unmarried. She had been in sex work for 2 years, part time, earning about Rs. 1,000 per client. Vanita also worked as a maid and went to film shootings. Her mother was also a sex worker (Sasita).

54 Vanni was 38 years old. She was married but lived alone. She had one child. Vanni had been a sex worker for 3 years, working part time. She did not do sex work during my fieldwork but worked in an export company.

55 Vasumathi was 38 years old. Vasumathi was forced to marry a man who had raped her. During their marriage, he was violent towards her and she had a divorce. At the time of my fieldwork she lived alone with her son. She had been in sex work for 9 years, but then stopped and worked as peer educator.

56 Zaima was about 50 years old. She was a Muslim. She was married with two children. She lived with her husband but also had female partners (she was the occasional partner of Komala). Zaima had been in sex work since she was 13. At the time of my research she occasionally still did sex work but predominantly pimped and worked as a counsellor in one of the NGOs, as well as in the film industry. Zaima's mother had also been a sex worker.

Bibliography

Abu-Lughod, L. (1990) 'The romance of resistance: tracing transformations of power through Bedouin women', *American Ethnologist*, 17(1): 41–55.

Agrawal, A. (2007) *Chaste Wives and Prostitute Sisters: Patriarchy and Prostitution among Bedias of India*. New Delhi: Routledge.

Ahmad, N. (2005) 'Trafficked persons or economic migrants? Bangladeshis in India', in Kempadoo, K., Sanghera, J. and Pattanaik, B. (eds) *Trafficking and Prostitution Reconsidered: New Perspectives on Migration, Sex Work and Human Rights*. Boulder, CO: Paradigm Publishers.

Amin, A. (2004) *Risk, Morality and Blame: a Critical Analysis of Government and U.S. Donor Responses to HIV Infections among Sex Workers in India*. Takoma Park, MD: Centre for Health and Gender Equity.

Anandhi, S. (1998) 'Reproductive bodies and regulated sexuality: birth control debates in early twentieth century Tamil Nadu', in John, M. and Nair, J. (eds) *A Question of Silence: the Sexual Economies of Modern India*. New Delhi: Kali for Women.

—— (2005) 'Sex and sensibility in Tamil politics', *Economic and Political Weekly*, 40: 4876–7.

AIDS Prevention and Control Society (APAC) (2003) *High Risk Behaviour Surveillance Survey in Tamil Nadu*, Wave VII. Chennai: AIDS Prevention and Control Project, Voluntary Health Services (VHS).

—— (2004) *HIV Risk Behaviour Surveillance Survey in Tamil Nadu*, Wave IX. Chennai: AIDS Prevention and Control Project, Voluntary Health Services, Chennai.

—— (2005a) *Prevalence of STI among Truckers and Helpers*. Chennai: AIDS Prevention and Control Project, Voluntary Health Services (VHS).

—— (2005b) *Prevalence of STI among Women in Prostitution*. Chennai: AIDS Prevention and Control Project, Voluntary Health Services (VHS).

Arunkumar, T. S., Irudaya Rajan, S. and Rakkee, T. (2004) 'HIV patients: knowledge and sexual behaviour patterns', *Economic and Political Weekly*, 39: 1208–10.

Asthana, S. and Oostvogels, R. (1996) 'Community participation in HIV prevention: problems and prospects for community-based strategies among female sex workers in Madras', *Social Science and Medicine*, 43: 133–48.

—— (2001) 'The social construction of male 'homosexuality' in India: implications for HIV transmission and preventions', *Social Science and Medicine*, 52: 707–21.

Barry, K. (1984) *Female Sexual Slavery*, New York: New York University Press.

Blanchard, J., O'Neil, J., Bhattacharjee, P., Orchard, T. and Moses, S. (2005) 'Understanding the social and cultural contexts of female sex workers in Karnataka, India: implication for prevention of HIV infection', *Journal of Infectious Diseases*, 191 (Suppl. 1): 139–46.

Boontinand, J. with Global Alliance Against Traffic in Women (2005) 'Feminist participatory action research in Mekong region', in Kempadoo, K., Sangher, J. and Pattanaik, B. (eds) *Trafficking and Prostitution Reconsidered: New Perspectives on Migration, Sex Work and Human Rights*. Boulder, CO: Paradigm Publishers.

Brahme, R. G., Sahay, S., Malhotra-Kohli, R., Divekar, A. D., Kharat, M. P., Risbud, A. R., Bollinger, R. C., Mehendale, S. M. and Paranjape, R. S. (2005) 'High-risk behaviour in young men attending sexually transmitting clinics in Pune', *AIDS Care*, 17: 377–85.

Brewis, J. and Linstead, S. (2000a) 'The worst thing is the screwing (1): consumption and management of identity in sex work', *Gender, Work and Organisation*, 7: 84–97.

—— (2000b) 'The worst thing is the screwing (2): context and career in sex work', *Gender, Work and Organisation*, 7: 168–80.

Busby, C. (2000) *The Performance of Gender: an Anthropology of Everyday Life in an Indian Fishing Village*. London: Athlone.

Caplan, P. (1985) *Class and Gender in India: a Study of Women and their Organizations in a South Indian City*. London: Tavistock.

Census (India) (2001) Migration tables, p. 18, Government of India. Available via: www.censusindia.net/results/dseries/data_highlights_D1D2D3.pdf (accessed 19 July 2007).

Census (Tamil Nadu) (2001) Government of Tamil Nadu statistics. Available via: www.tn.gov.in/economy/eco-oct2001-12.htm> (accessed 19 July 2007).

Chatterjee, P. (1989) 'The nationalist resolution of the women's question', in Sangari, K. and Vaid, S. (eds) *Recasting Women: Essays in Colonial History*. New Delhi: Kali for Women.

Cohen, L. (2005) 'Kothi wars: AIDS cosmopolitanism and the morality of classification', in Adams, V. and Pigg, S. L. (eds) *Sex in Development: Science, Sexuality, and Morality in Global Perspective*. Durham, NC: Duke University Press.

Cornish, F. (2006) 'Empowerment to participate: a case study of participation by Indian sex workers in HIV prevention', *Journal of Community and Applied Social Psychology*, 16: 301–15.

Cusick, L. (1998) 'Non-use of condoms of prostitute women', *AIDS Care*, 10: 133–46.

Dandona, L., Sisodia, P., Kumar, P., Ramesh, Y. K., Kumar, A., Rao, C., Marseille, E., Someshwar, M., Marshall, N. and Kahn, J. (2005) 'HIV prevention programmes for female sex workers in Andhra Pradesh, India: outputs, cost and efficiency', *BMC Public Health*, 5(98). Available via: www.biomedcentral.com/1471-2458/1475/1498 (accessed 31 January 2009).

Das, V. (1975) 'Marriage among Hindus', in Jain, D. (ed.) *Indian Women*, New Delhi: Government of India.

Day, S. (2007) *On the Game: Women and Sex Work*. London: Pluto Press.

Deliege, R. (1992) 'Replication and consensus: untouchability, caste and ideology in India', *Man, New Series*, 27(1): 155–73.

Dell, H. (2005) 'Ordinary sex, prostitutes and middle–class wives: liberalisation and national identity in India', in Adams, V. and Pigg, S. L. (eds) *Sex in Development. Science, Sexuality and Morality in Global Perspective*. Durham and London: Duke University Press.

Dickey, S. (1993) 'The politics of adulation: cinema and the reproduction of politicians in South India', *Journal of South Asian Studies*, 52: 340–72.

Dyson, T. and Moore, M. (1983) 'On kinship structure, female autonomy and demographic behaviour in India', *Population and Development Review*, 9(1): 35–60.

Egnor, M. (1980) 'On the meaning of *sakti* to women in Tamil Nadu', in Wadley, S. S. (ed.) *The Powers of Tamil Women*, Syracuse, New York: Maxwell School of Citizenship and Public Affairs, Syracuse University.

Evans, C. and Lambert, H. (1997) 'Health-seeking strategies and sexual health among female sex workers in urban India: implications for research and service provision', *Social Science and Medicine*, 44: 1791–803.

Evans, K. (1998) 'Contemporary *devadasis*: empowered auspicious women or exploited prostitutes?', *Bulletin of the John Rylands University Library of Manchester*, 80: 23–38.

Forrester, D. (1976) 'Factions and film stars: Tamil Nadu politics since 1971', *Asian Survey*, 16: 283–96.

Foucault, M. (1998 [1976]) *History of Sexuality*, vol. 1. London: Penguin.

Fredrick, J. (2005) 'The myth of Nepal-to-India sex trafficking: its creation, its maintenance, and its influence on anti-trafficking interventions', in Kempadoo, K., Sangher, J. and Pattanaik, B. (eds) *Trafficking and Prostitution Reconsidered: New Perspectives on Migration, Sex Work and Human Rights*. Boulder, CO: Paradigm Publisher.

Geetha, V. (1998) 'On bodily hurt and love', in John, M. and Nair, J. (eds) *A Question of Silence: the Sexual Economies of Modern India*. New Delhi: Kali for Women.

George, G. (2003) 'Pineapples and oranges, Brahmins and Sudras: Periyar feminists and narratives of gender and regional identity in South India', *Anthropologica*, 45: 265–81.

Ghosh, S. (2004) 'The shadow lines of citizenship: prostitutes struggles over workers' rights', *Identity, Culture and Politics*, 5(1&2): 105–23.

Gisselquist, D. and Correa, M. (2006) 'How much does heterosexual commercial sex contribute to India's HIV epidemic?', *International Journal of STD and AIDS*, 17: 736–42.

Go, V., Johnson, S., Bentley, M., Sivaram, S., Srikrishnan, A., Solomon, S. and Celentano, D. (2003) 'When HIV-prevention messages and gender norms clash: the impact of domestic violence on women's HIV risk in slums of Chennai', *AIDS and Behaviour*, 7: 263–72.

Goffman, E. (1968) *Stigma: Notes on the Management of Spoiled Identity*. London: Penguin.

Gooptu, N. (2000) 'Sex workers in Calcutta and the dynamics of collective action: political activism, community identity and group behaviour', Working papers No. 185. Helsinki: The United Nations University, WIDER (World Institute for Development Economics Research).

Gorringe, H. (2005) *Untouchable Citizens: Dalit Movements and Democratization in Tamil Nadu*. New Delhi: Sage Publications.

—— (2006) 'Establishing territory: the spatial bases and practices of the DPI', in De Neeve, G.and Donner, H. (eds) *The Meaning of the Local: Politics of Place in Urban India*. Oxon: Routledge.

Hancock, M. E. (1999) *Womanhood in the Making: Domestic Ritual and Public Culture in Urban South India*. Boulder, CO: Westview Press.

Hart, G. and Barnard, M. (2003) 'Jump on top, get the job done: strategies employed by female prostitutes to reduce the risk of client violence', in Stanko, E. A. (eds) *The Meanings of Violence*. London: Routledge.

Hershman, P. (1974) 'Hair, sex and dirt', *Man*, 9: 274–98.

Immoral Traffic (Prevention) Act (ITPA) (1956) Government of India.

Jayasree, A. K. (2004) 'Searching for justice for body and self in a coercive environment: sex work in Kerala, India', *Reproductive Health Matters*, 12: 58–67.

Jeffery, P. (1979) *Frogs in a Well: Indian Women in Purdah*. London: Zed Press.

—— (1998) 'Agency, activism and agendas', in Jeffery, P. and Basu, A. (eds) *Appropriating Gender: Women's Activism and Politicized Religion in South Asia*, New York: London: Routledge.

Jeffery, P. and Jeffery, R. (1996) *Don't Marry Me to a Plowman!: women's everyday lives in rural North India*. Boulder, CO: Westview Press.

Jeffery, P., Jeffery, R. and Lyon, A. (1989) *Labour Pains and Labour Power: women and childbearing in India*. London: Zed.

Jeffery, P., Jeffery, R. and Rao, M (2007) 'Safe motherhood initiatives: contributions from small-scale studies', *Indian Journal of Gender Studies*, 14: 285–94.

Jeffreys, S. (1997) *The Idea of Prostitution*. North Melbourne: Spinifex.

John, M. and Nair, J. (eds) *A Question of Silence: the Sexual Economies of Modern India*. New Delhi: Kali for Women.

Kapadia, K. (ed.) (2002) *The Violence of Development: the Politics of Identity, Gender and Social Inequalities in India*. New Delhi: Kali for Women.

Karnik, N. (2001) 'Locating HIV/AIDS in India: cautionary notes on the globalization of categories', *Science, Technology and Human Values*, 26: 321–48.

Kempadoo, K. and Doezema, J. (1998) *Global Sex Workers: Rights, Resistance, and Redefinition*. New York: London: Routledge.

Kersenboom-Story, S. (1987) *Nitysuamangali: Devadasi Tradition in South India*. Delhi: Motila Banarsidass.

Kishwar, M. (1986) 'Gandhi on women', *Race and Class*, 28(1): 43–61.

—— (1999) *Off the Beaten Track: Rethinking Gender Justice for Indian Women*. New Delhi: Oxford University Press.

Kulkarni, V., Kulkarni, S. and Spaeth, K. (2004) 'Men who have sex with men: a study in urban western Maharashtra', in Verma, R., Pelto, P., Schensun, S. and

Joshi, A. (eds) *Sexuality in the Time of AIDS: Contemporary Perspectives from Communities in India*. New Delhi: Sage.

Laukamm-Josten U., Mwizarubi B. K., Outwater A., Mwaijonga C. L., Valadez J. J., Nyamwaya D., Swai R., Saidel T. and Nyamuryekung'e K. (2000) 'Preventing HIV infection through peer education and condom promotion among truck drivers and their sexual partners in Tanzania, 1990–1993', *AIDS Care*, 12(1): 27–41.

MacKeganey, N. P. and Barnard, M. (1996) *Sex Work on the Streets: Prostitutes and their Clients*. Buckingham, PA: Open University Press.

MacPhail, C. and Campbell, C. (2001) 'I think condoms are good but, aai, I hate those things: condom use among adolescents and young people in a Southern African township,' *Social Science and Medicine*, 52: 1613–27.

Mahmood, S. (2005) *Politics of Piety: the Islamic Revival and the Feminist Subject*. Princeton, NJ: Princeton University Press.

Moghadam, V. M. (2005) *Globalizing Women: Transnational Feminist Networks*. Baltimore, MD: Johns Hopkins University Press.

Moody, P. (2002) 'Kidnapping, elopement and abduction: an ethnography of love marriage in Delhi', in Orsini, F. (ed.) *Love in South Asia*, Cambridge: Cambridge University Press.

Mosse, D. (2005) *Cultivating Development: an Ethnography of Aid Policy and Practice*. London: Pluto Press.

Murray, A. and Robinson, T. (1996) 'Minding your peers and queers: female sex workers in the AIDS discourse in Australia and South-east Asia', *Gender, Place and Culture*, 3(1): 43–59.

NACO (2004) *Annual Report 2002–2004*. National AIDS Control Organisation, Ministry of Health and Family Welfare, Government of India.

NACO (2007) *Targeted Interventions under NACP3. Operationalised guidelines. Vol. 1. Core High Risk Groups*, National AIDS Control Organisation, Ministry of Health and Family Welfare, Government of India.

Nag, M. (2001) 'Anthropological perspectives on prostitution and AIDS in India', *Economic and Political Weekly*, 36: 4025–30.

Nagle, J. (1997) *Whores and Other Feminists*. New York: London: Routledge.

Nencel, L. (2001) *Ethnography and Prostitution in Peru*. Sterling: Pluto Press.

Nencel, L. (2005) 'Feeling gender speak: intersubjectivity and fieldwork practice with women who prostitute in Lima, Peru', *European Journal of Women's Studies*, 12: 345–61.

Oldenburg, V. (1990) 'Lifestyle as resistance: the case of the courtesans of Lucknow, India', *Feminist Studies*, 16: 259–87.

O'Neil, J., Orchard, T., Swarankar, R. C., Blanchard, J., Gurav, K. and Moses, S. (2004) 'Dhanda, dharma and disease: traditional sex work and HIV/AIDS in rural India', *Social Science and Medicine*, 59: 851–60.

Ong, A and Collier, S. (2005) *Global Assemblages: Technology, Politics and Ethics as Anthropological Problems*. Oxford: Blackwell Publishing.

Orr, L. C. (2000) *Donors, Devotees, and Daughters of God: Temple Women in Medieval Tamil Nadu*. New York: Oxford University Press.

Pallikavadath, S., Sanneh, A., McWhirter, J. and Stones, W. (2005) 'Rural women's knowledge of AIDS in higher prevalence states of India: reproductive health and socio-cultural correlates', *Health Promotion International*, 20: 249–59.

Pandian, M. S. S. (1992) *The Image Trap: M.G. Ramachandran in Film and Politics*. New Delhi: Sage.

Pardasani, M. (2005) 'HIV prevention and sex workers: an international lesson in empowerment', *International Journal of Social Welfare*, 14: 116–26.

Patel, S. (1988) 'Construction and reconstruction of woman in Gandhi', *Economic and Political Weekly*, 20 February: 377–86.

Pheterson, G. and St. James, M. (1989) *A Vindication of the Rights of Whores*, Seattle, WA: Seal Press.

Puri, J. (1999) *Woman, Body, Desire in Post-colonial India: Narratives of Gender and Sexuality*. New York: London: Routledge.

Raj, S. (1993) *Prostitution in Madras: a Study in Historical Perspective*. Delhi: Konark Publications.

Rao, V., Gupta, I., Lokshin, M. and Jana, S. (2003) 'Sex workers and the cost of safe sex: compensating differential for condom use among Calcutta sex workers', *Journal of Development Economics*, 71: 585–603.

Raymond, J. (1998) 'Prostitution as violence against women: NGO stonewalling in Bejing and elsewhere', *Women's Studies International Forum*, 21(1): 1–9.

Reddy, G. (2004) 'Crossing lines of subjectivity: the negotiation of sexual identity in Hyderabad, India', in Srivastava, S. (ed.) *Sexual Sites, Seminal Attitudes: Sexualities, Masculinities and Culture in South Asia*. New Delhi: Sage.

—— (2005a) *With Respect to Sex. Negotiating Hijra Identity in South India*. Chicago: University of Chicago Press.

—— (2005b) 'Geographies of Contagion: *Hijras, Kothis* and the Politics of Sexual Marginality in Hyderabad', *Anthropology and Medicine*, 12: 255–70.

Reynolds, H. (1980) 'The auspicious married woman', in Wadley, S. S. (ed.) *The Powers of Tamil Women*. Syracuse, New York: Maxwell School of Citizenship and Public Affairs, Syracuse University.

Rogers, M. (2007) 'Between fantasy and "reality": Tamil film star fan club networks and the political economy of film fandom', presented at the Edinburgh South Asia Seminar Series, University of Edinburgh, 22 March 2007.

Sanders, T. (2005a) 'It's just acting: sex workers: strategies for capitalising on sexuality', *Gender, Work and Organisation*, 12: 319–42.

—— (2005b) *Sex Work: a Risky Business*. Cullompton, Devon: Willan.

Sariola, S. and Simpson, R. (2008) 'The medical, the bioethical and the rhetorical: reflections on international health initiatives in Sri Lanka and India', presented at the South Asia Anthropology Group Conference, University of Durham, 8–9 September 2008.

Scott, J. C. (1985) *Weapons of the Weak: Everyday Forms of Peasant Resistance*. New Haven, CT: Yale University Press.

Seidel, G. (1993) 'The competing discourses on HIV/AIDS in Sub-Saharan Africa: discourses of rights and empowerment vs. discourses of control and exclusion', *Social Science and Medicine*, 36: 175–94.

Sivaram, S., Aylur, K., Srikrishnan, A., Latkin, C., Johnson, S., Go, V., Bentley, M., Solomon, S. and Celentano, D. (2004a) 'Development of an opinion leader-led HIV prevention intervention among alcohol users in Chennai, India', *AIDS Education and Prevention*, 16: 137–49.

Sivaram, S., Lakshmi, S., Go, V., Srikrishnan, A. K., Celentano, D., Solomon, S. and Bentley, M. (2004b) 'Telling stories: narrative scenarios to assess sexual norms for an HIV prevention study in Chennai, India', in Verma, R., Pelto, P., Schensun, S. and Joshi, A. (eds) *Sexuality in the Time of AIDS: Contemporary Perspectives from Communities in India*. New Delhi: Sage.

Sivaram, S., Johnsson, S., Bentley, M., Go, V., Latkin, C., Srikrishnan, A., Celentano, D. and Solomon, S. (2005) 'Sexual health promotion in Chennai, India: key role of communication among social networks', *Health Promotion International*, 20: 327–33.

Sleightholme, C. and Sinha, I. (2002) *Guilty without Trial: Women in the Sex Trade in Calcutta*. Calcutta: Stree.

Srivastava, S. (2004) 'Non-Gandhian sexuality, commodity cultures and a 'happy married life': masculine and sexual cultures in the metropolis', in Srivastava, S. (ed.) *Sexual Sites, Seminal Attitudes: Sexualities, Masculinities and Culture in South Asia*. New Delhi: Sage.

Steinbrook, R. (2007) 'HIV in India: a complex topic', *New England Journal of Medicine*, 356: 1089–93.

Subadra (1999) 'Violence against women: wife battering in Chennai', *Economic and Political Weekly*, 34: 28–33.

Sundaram, K. and Tendulkar, S. (2003) 'Poverty among social and economic groups in India in 1990s', *Economic and Political Weekly*, 38: 5263–76.

Sundari Ravindran, T. K. (1999) 'Women's autonomy in Tamil Nadu', *Economic and Political Weekly*, 34: 34–44.

Swaminathan, P. (2002) 'The violence of gender-based development: going beyond social and demographic indicators', in Kapadia, K. (ed.) *The Violence of Development: Politics of Identity, Gender and Social Inequalities in India*. New Delhi: Kali for Women.

—— (2004) 'The trauma of 'wage employment' and the burden of work for women in India: evidences and experiences', Working paper no. 186, Madras Institution of Development Studies, pp. 3–36.

Tambiah, Y. (2005) 'Turncoat bodies: sexuality and sex work under militarization in Sri Lanka', *Gender and Society*, 19: 243–61.

Trawick, M. (1990) *Notes on Love in a Tamil Family*. Berkeley, CA: University of California Press.

Treichler, P. A. (1999) *How to Have Theory in an Epidemic: cultural chronicles of AIDS*, Durham, NC: Duke University Press.

United Nations Joint Programme on HIV/AIDS (UNAIDS) (2006) Fact sheet 06: Asia. Geneva: UNAIDS. Available via: http://data.unaids.org/pub/GlobalReport/2006/200605–FS_Asia_en.pdf (accessed 27 February 2009).

—— (2007) '2.5 million people in India living with HIV, according to new estimates', press release. Available via: http://data.unaids.org/pub/PressRelease/2007/070706_indiapressrelease_en.pdf (accessed 27 February 2009).

Van Hollen, C. C. (2003) *Birth on the Threshold: Childbirth and Modernity in South India*. New Delhi: Zubaan.

Van Raay, C. (2006) *God's Callgirl*. London: Ebury Press.

Venkataramana, C. B. S. and Sarada, P. V. (2001) 'Extent and speed of spread of HIV infection in India through the commercial sex networks: a perspective', *Tropical Medicine and International Health*, 6: 1040–61.

Vera-Sanso, P. (2006) 'Conformity and contestation: social heterogeneity in south Indian settlements', in De Neeve, G. and Donner, H. (eds) *The Meaning of the Local: Politics of Place in Urban India*. Oxon: Routledge.

Verma, R. and Lhungdim, H. (2004) 'Sexuality and sexual behaviours in rural India: evidence from a five state study', in Verma, R., Pelto, P., Schensun, S. and Joshi, A. (eds) *Sexuality in the Time of AIDS: Contemporary Perspectives from Communities in India*, New Delhi: Sage.

Viramma, Racine, J. and Racine, J. L. (1997) *Viramma: Life of an Untouchable.* London: Verso.

Visvanathan, S. (2006) 'Men in a muddle: An Exclusive Sex Survey', *India Today*, 45: 37–76.

Wadley, S. S. (1980a) *The Powers of Tamil Women*. Syracuse, NY: Maxwell School of Citizenship and Public Affairs, Syracuse University.

—— (1980b) 'The paradoxical powers of Tamil women', in Wadley, S. S. (ed.) *The Powers of Tamil Women*, Syracuse, New York: Maxwell School of Citizenship and Public Affairs, Syracuse University.

Wardlow, H. (2004) 'Anger, economy and female agency: problematizing "prostitution" and "sex work" among Hull in Papua New Guinea', *Journal of Women in Culture and Society*, 29: 1017–40.

Wardlow, H. (2006) *Wayward Women: Sexuality and Agency in New Guinea Society*. Berkeley, CA: University of California Press.

Zatz, N. (1997) 'Sex work/Sex act: law, labour, and desire in constructions of prostitution', *Signs: Journal of Women in Culture and Society*, 22: 277–308.

Other websites and web-based sources that are mentioned in this book

APAC NGOs. Available via: www.apacvhs.org/NP_APAC_NGOs.html (accessed 31 July 2007).

CAPACS NGOs. Available via: www.capacs.org/ngos.htm (accessed 31 July 2007).

The Hindu, 30 May 2007. Available via: www.hindu.com/2007/05/30/stories/2007053015260300.htm (accessed 26 June 2007).

NACO and Phase 2 of HIV prevention. Available via: www.nacoonline.org/abt_phase2.htm (accessed 22 October 2006).

TAI project. Available via: www.taivhs.org/about.htm (accessed 21 October 2008).

UNAIDS and HIV prevention policies. Available via: www.unaids.org/en/Policies/HIV_Prevention/default.asp (accessed 13 August 2007).

Index